WHAT TO EXPECT WHEN YOU ARE EXPECTING CANCER

A STAGE IVB THROAT CANCER SURVIVOR SPEAKS OF LIFE; BEFORE, DURING & BEYOND CANCER

D. J. Paulsen

ISBN:1492387789
ISBN-13:9781492387787

DEDICATION

Dedicated to all the survivors out there and in loving memory of Elsie
Belle Bush Sweet and Richard Theodore Sweet.

CONTENTS

ACKNOWLEDGMENTS

I would like to say thank you to Winship Cancer Center Atlanta Ga. and an extra special thanks to Dr. B., my husband and my kids David, Tennille and Kristina and Megan... who made sure I survived to write this.

SECTION I: LIFE BEFORE CANCER

1 GET PRO ACTIVE DOING THE DOCTOR SCENE

Have you, a friend or a loved one, ever felt like you were trapped on a medical merry go round of seemingly endless trips to countless specialists and doctors? Have you ever felt like you were being forced to stay on the ride and endure going around and around from test to test, trying this prescription pill or that one in search of relief without success because you knew something was wrong and needed to know why you did not feel well? I have been there done that and then some. Doing the Doctor Scene is for everyone, with or without cancer. The tips and advice within this chapter are geared towards being more pro-active in our own health care, about making sure at your next doctor's appointment the test results you have waited for, even if they are not what you wanted to hear, are at least accurate, and making sure important clues about your health have not been overlooked.

At my life's midway point I was pretty much cruising along, I certainly was not losing any sleep considering the possibility of developing cancer. I have always been one of those active individuals, enjoying competitive sports and outdoor activities, whether softball games on the grass or trying to ski in the snow (Notice I said try? There is a hysterical story there and I smile reminiscing). I was known to ride anything, from jumping on a horse or a motorcycle to an ATV or a snowmobile. If it was outdoors and fun I was there. I lived most of my life true to my country roots, fairly quietly away from big cities, with my family, animals, gardens and nature around about me. Mind you staying in the country was not always without some protest over the years from my four children as they grew up. They loved being out in the country when they were little, but each one in their own time, as they grew older, entering High School, bemoaned "being in the boonies"… Talk about full circle, now that they are grown and they are parents, Grandma's place in the boonies is much beloved again by all… but wait I digress. Anyway here I was with life stretched out before me, the nest was empty and I had time and freedom to do whatever I wanted, as opposed to doing what was needed, more than I had ever experienced in all of my life. Believe it or not it is not as easy adjusting to free time as one may think. I had gotten the hang of it though, becoming involved with a number of volunteer programs, continuing my work in the construction business which was going good, and I was also enjoying a rebirth of passion and interest in art and writing. It was just when I was about ready to start patting myself on the back, thinking I was aging pretty well for a baby boomer with a kid up into his thirties… that I started to not feel well.

I have never been one to run to the doctor for every little thing, I mean the kids had their pediatrician of course, but quite frankly delivering four kids C-Section had been pretty much the extent of my experience and close relationships with hospitals or primary care physicians. Appointments with the Doctor's office became harder and harder to avoid making though. Joint pains and extreme fatigue, which I had chalked up to over exertion and just plain getting older, not *old* mind you, just *older*, refused to resolve over time on their own. Headaches became more frequent and severe. Finally I was forced to call and make an appointment. This began a round of tests and visits to specialists in various fields that without exaggeration lasted over 4 years. It was a period of time during which I lost weight and muscle mass, most of my hair, financial stability, and a lot of my faith in the medical profession; this was long before eventually being diagnosed with cancer at a very advanced stage IVB.

What I noticed and found very frustrating right off the bat in my search for answers, which originated at my primary care physician's office all those years ago, eventually spreading to include countless other specialists, such as but not limited to rheumatologists, gastroenterologists, and even neurologists, was that at each appointment, regardless of symptoms or complaints, the doctors would all offer one new pill or another that they felt I "Just had to try". This was without ever giving or offering any actual diagnosis. I mean how do you prescribe a pill without a diagnosis?

IF YOU HAVE BEEN GIVEN A PRESCRIPTION FOR A MEDICATION BUT NOT A DIAGNOSIS QUESTION YOUR DOCTOR FURTHER.

I also learned that generally these pills were often coincidently involved in strong marketing pushes, the latest pharmaceutical wonder currently or soon to be featured in the latest colorful enticing commercial on a television screen near you. Even worse was the fact that more often than not these medications were not even related to the symptoms that were being presented with. Also they were accompanied by lengthy lists of possible side effects. Generally these warning labels were longer and far scarier, describing worse symptoms than the initial reason that prompted the office visit. Hmm, let me consider, would I rather deal with my knees being a bit stiff and occasional headaches or possible complications such as heart arrhythmias, breathing difficulties, suicidal thoughts, or anal leakage?

I was becoming increasingly dissatisfied with the listening skills and bedside manners of the physicians I saw. I didn't even want to go to any more doctors at all. Early on the doctors claimed I had fibromyalgia, even though I did not have the key pressure point symptoms. Fibromyalgia, while a real condition, basically became a doctor's catchall diagnosis from the late 1990's onward, whenever they didn't have an obvious reason what was wrong, it was a good excuse to offer the latest new wonder pill to a New Guinea pig / patient. I remember an episode after one of my appointments; I had been having headaches and joint pain at the time, and after waiting two months for the problems to resolve again on their own I gave in and called to schedule a visit. I was prescribed a "new" pill, which upon research I learned like many of these other *miracle medications* came up under the classification of anti depressant. Due to copy right laws I cannot name these medications here. It was not long before I called the office, complaining to the doctor's nurse that the pill prescribed had made me feel horrible. I was jittery and grinding my teeth, finding myself walking in circles, couldn't sit, couldn't stay up, couldn't eat or sleep or even poop properly for crying out loud. She did actually return my call, and I was told to "Go ahead and *double* the dose and *give it a couple of weeks*". Seriously?

ONLY YOU KNOW YOUR BODY, DO NOT BE AFRAID TO BE PERSISTANT AND INSISTANT WITH YOUR DOCTOR IF YOU FEEL SOMETHING IS WRONG.

Without exaggeration I have a box with these "wonder pill" prescription bottles that were suggested by physicians. Even though I had reached a point going in for the appointments where I told the doctors "I do not want any anti depressants", and they would say "oh they are not", upon research all proved to be classed as anti depressants and after I had caught on these all remained unused. For an individual suffering from a true depression disorder, a condition which is often associated with chemical imbalances in the brain, these prescriptions and others in the same class of anti depressants may offer relief of symptoms; but as I tried to tell the doctors, and I can tell you from personal experience, when prescribed for a person like myself who is not depressed, anti depressants can cause an individual to experience severe and completely unnecessary adverse reactions. Also, once there is mention in your medical history of being prescribed these drugs to treat your nonexistent "depression" it can be very difficult to get a doctor to really listen to you as you are explaining your symptoms.

DO NOT ACCEPT ANTI-DEPRESSANTS WHEN PRESCRIBED IN ABSENCE OF A TRUE DEPRESSIVE DISORDER, THESE MAY CREATE ADDITIONAL, UNNECESSARY, AND

SOMETIMES DANGEROUS NEW SYMPTOMS, AS WELL AS POSSIBLY MASK TRUE SYMPTOMS OF AN UNDER LYING DISORDER.

My relationship with my primary care physicians became almost antagonistic. I tried switching to different physicians, looking for one who would *listen*. I had been trying to find answers for so long like I said I had reached the point in the examining room I was telling the doctor "and NO, I don't want the newest anti-depressant". It is amazing the number of prescription bottles one can accumulate in the course of trying to find answers to why you're not feeling well, I mean really I told them I would be looking it up and would not be taking it if I found it was being prescribed off label and was intended as an anti depressant. These new *progressive* drugs are so freely and readily prescribed. This practice of here's a pill is in my humble opinion a direct result of kick backs and agreements between the drug manufacturers and healthcare providers that are intended to enable the pharmaceutical corporations to compile the desired clinical *empirical* statistics required to meet FDA standards. This practice of off label prescribing has recently gained some slight main stream media attention, but demands much more attention than it is receiving. Change may come some day, but currently anti depressants are all too often first choice to treat vague symptoms, and are prescribed for "off label" use by primary care physicians far too often in my humble opinion and experience. Even worse, this overly prescribed class of drugs can mask existing symptoms, as well as result in the development of new symptoms and health concerns.

RESEARCH WHAT YOUR DOCTOR PRESCRIBES, IF YOU FEEL MEDICATIONS ARE BEING PRESCRIBED FOR DEPRESSION AND ARE NOT SUITABLE AND DO NOT APPLY TO YOU HAVE THESE CONCERNS OFFICIALLY NOTED IN YOUR MEDICAL HISTORY FILE.

Yet another very important lesson learned at a cost through my personal experience in the course of seeking treatment that I had not even considered early on, but I now know to be a possibility, out of the norm blood work test results do get overlooked. I know because it happened to me, and not just on one occasion. If I had thought of requesting a copy of my lab reports it is possible that my cancer may have been detected earlier, maybe not. I of course in hind sight cannot be sure of that, but seriously how hard is it to look over results carefully? Trust me you should request a copy and look over lab test results yourself. If the doctor's staff looks at you a little weird the first time or two you ask for copies don't worry about it, they'll get used to you asking and get over it.

GET INTO THE HABIT OF ALWAYS REQUESTING A COPY OF YOUR RESULTS EVERY TIME TESTS ARE DONE, DO NOT RELY ON OTHERS EYES.

Like I said I was surprised to learn these clearly marked results were missed. Out of the norm results are generally highlighted in bold print. Additionally there may be a plus or minus symbol as well or instead of. There may be a letter symbol such as H (high) or L (low) used to indicate excessive or decreased values out of the normal range.

WE WOULD NO DOUBT BE SHOCKED IF THERE WAS AN ACCURATE METHOD TO CALCULATE WHAT SHOULD BE CONSIDERED RED FLAG BLOOD TEST RESULTS THAT ARE OVERLOOKED OR MISSED. THIS WOULD BE DIFFICULT TO DETERMINE THOUGH, BECAUSE HOW WOULD YOU COUNT SOMETHING THAT IS MISSED, UNLESS YOU FOUND IT?

It was on one of my last few visits, just prior to my official cancer diagnosis, that my primary doctor was looking over my chart and asked me "what did you do as far as follow up on the highly elevated calcium and muscle enzyme levels from last year"? Well gee, since no one had ever informed me last year that they were elevated, what would I have done? This would have been that same year, while those calcium levels were up, that I was referred to a cardiac specialist because of an episode of chest pains, and abnormal EKG results. I myself did not learn until much, much later that calcium levels in the body are very strictly regulated, with a small window of *normal*. I did not know that elevated calcium levels could cause heart problems. The doctors should have though. They not only missed the lab results, but when the high calcium affected my heart, they did not recheck lab results, or do further blood test. They chose to treat a symptom, and passed me on to the heart specialist. This doctor did not check calcium levels, no doubt because he would have expected that this was done by my primary before I was sent to him. Which ironically it was; but somehow those results were overlooked. I was seeing the cardiac doctor for almost six months. This of course included more tests, lost time from work and money. The first few visits EKG testing had the cardiac doctor concerned as well, but, with weeks between visits, eventually my heart rhythms settled back into normal patterns. I was again left with no answers for the extreme fatigue or muscle and joint pains, or the headaches after all of the time and insurance dollars invested. A total of six months was spent going to appointments for ultrasounds, stress tests and MRI's, and follow ups because of that one missed out of norm test. What was the end result? My heart was given a clean bill of health, and I was again left on my own to wonder "what is wrong with me?"

The elevated calcium levels, which I now know can affect heart function, were most likely an early clue from the parathyroid glands that something was wrong. This response was probably triggered in the parathyroid glands due to invasion by the progressing encroachment of the silent throat cancer. Most likely what happened was a period of over activity (high calcium blood levels) from the parathyroids, followed by under activity due to advancement and constriction due to growth of the tumor. My heart, relieved of the burden caused by the excess calcium levels, had returned to its normal function. While the cardiac testing that was done did assure me that my heart was actually quite strong and healthy, I feel this was an early cancer detection window of opportunity that was missed.

Calcium levels being out of the normal range happened to be a very important clue. Any fluctuations out of the accepted very narrow scale of accepted normal could be indicative of very serious health concerns…such as cancer. I had even called the office for those results too, because over two weeks had passed and there had been no return call in the 2-3 days as promised. I had been told they would definitely be contacting me, because of the continued elevation in muscle enzymes from previous testing. There was *supposed* to be a call back to tell me if these levels were up, down or the same. When I called them, and finally did get the nurse on the line she said the muscle enzymes *were* still elevated, but that everything else had checked out fine.

I was pretty incredulous at the time, because I was going through a rough patch at that point, and really didn't feel well. So I made one more appointment. That was the visit with the whacky EKG that sent me off to the cardiac doctor. I have also forgotten to mention the vascular specialist I went to at some point along the way in that long line of doctors who had the opportunity to check me over. I was sent there because my primary doctor while I was complaining about the recurring headaches, after listening with a stethoscope along the side of my neck, felt carotid artery blockages could be a cause. That doctor was a complete waste of months of time and money. He did say after testing that my left side was ninety percent blocked. I was made to come in for appointments once a month. Every time I came in they would ultrasound the arteries in my neck, and say yep, still blocked, and make me another appointment. At each appointment I was lectured and told my carotids were blocked because I was a smoker, and essentially my health was my own fault. My patience with this particular doctor wore so thin that I finally lost it and demanded answers. It did not end well. That doctor's office was one of three over the course of searching for answers to my very real health concerns that I was actually thrown out of and told do not come back. Yes, that really happens. His office does have the distinction of being the only to threaten to call the police on me though, because I refused to leave until provided copies of my records. The other two were more polite when we decided to part ways. Our conversation was more along the lines of if I did not want to take what they prescribed then they saw no point in continuing the doctor patient relationship. To which of course, I had to agree. I mean really if all they were going to do was prescribe anti depressants that I wasn't going to take because they made me feel even worse, yes, they were right, there was no point coming back. One was a new primary care physician I had switched to and the other was a rheumatologist.

At the last pre diagnosis appointment I was told by my primary that they had checked everything they could think of to check, and that all labs were now normal, except for the still elevated muscle enzymes. I was given the *latest* miracle medicine, this was another well known name brand that copyright restrictions would necessitate permission to use their name, this one started with the letter S. It was strongly recommended by my physician that I give it a try, for at least two months. In frustration I again temporarily gave up trying to find answers in a doctor's office.

REMEMBER IF YOU KNOW SOMETHING IS WRONG, DON'T BE AFRAID TO BE PERSISTENT.

I wish I had been more persistent myself, but it was frustrating to hear time and again they could find nothing wrong, and being treated like it was either my own faulty or it was all in my head, like I was being a hypochondriac that needed to be on pills. This frustration with the medical profession probably played a role in why I was one of those people who thought I could never get cancer. Gosh, if I ever got cancer that would mean I needed to trust a doctor, and by that point in my life, that just wasn't happening. The day I would meet my oncology team, who I did learn to trust, was still months away, and would not happen until after I had completely lost my voice.

I personally came to feel that too many doctors were not and would not really listen unless or until they had something obvious and concrete staring them in the face. It seemed they no longer wanted to work to find the answers to health questions. Wouldn't it be nice if art always mimicked life? Then we would have more physicians like the doctors on television shows that so dramatically and aggressively tackle and solve all sorts of medical conditions. Rather than look for the cause of problems, before they reach a point of being debilitating or deadly, which should be what a primary care doctor is supposed to do, all too often they try first to treat the symptoms as they appear. This tends to hold true until or unless there is a red flag warning symptom so far outside the normal range that it cannot be ignored. For example lab results (that are not overlooked), new unexplained lumps, bumps or discolorations that they can see and touch, easy to spot vital sign distress signals like blood pressure or heart rhythm irregularities, severe pain, or, like in my case completely losing my voice. If you have nothing that is *obvious* then you must be depressed. Here's your pill.

After so many frustrating office visits for vague come and go symptoms without definitive answers I think a lot of people do like I did. We just quit going. Maybe when we give up going to doctors, we give up worrying about what may be wrong? I know that I had reached a point I told my husband "That's it, until something gets bad enough to send me to the emergency room; I'm just not going anymore."

In defense of doctors, I know my personal experience has biased my opinion, I feel it fair I must add I am quite sure there are still a few good primary care practices that are well staffed, well organized, compassionate and conscientious.

2 GAME OF CHANCE: WHO WILL GET CANCER AND WHO WILL NOT?

A Game of Chance discusses various commonly known risk factors, as well as a few lesser known possible contributing factors, which have been associated with the development of different types of cancers. Is anyone really more at risk than the next person? Or is it an even playing field? Does it help to worry in advance about cancer or are we more at risk if we don't worry about it? To all of these questions there are yes and no answers to be found in that old adage about everything in moderation, including moderation (Oscar Wilde). Shall we examine some of the possibilities?

There have been multiple studies regarding the effects on the body from excessive worrying and stress that strongly suggest that there exist a correlation between stress and physical ailments. Does this mean someone who worries a lot about possibly getting cancer will get cancer because of worrying about it specifically? I don't think so. While there are people who do worry excessively about getting cancer, the dreaded big C, you must keep in mind that they are most likely worriers about many aspects of their lives. Some people are born worriers, it's not a flaw. Worriers are people like Moms and best friends, the husband working and planning for his family's financial future, worriers can be anyone. Funny thing is, I am a worrier, I just never worried about getting cancer.

Often it is a specific event that will set a worrier off to becoming overly concerned about getting cancer. Someone close to them may have or had cancer in the past. Maybe concerns about certain environmental exposures indigenous to their personal situation, or even reading a lot on the topic via the internet while researching symptoms, all can fuel a worrier's fears. So, while they may worry about getting cancer, I do not feel it would be directly caused due to worrying about developing cancer that made them ill. I would have to say if worry was found to be a cause of cancer then it would no doubt be a culmination of many worries, not just worrying about getting cancer.

MENTAL STATE OF HEALTH, HAPPINESS AND STABILITY CAN PLAY A ROLE IN KEEPING YOUR BODY HEALTHY.

It may be difficult for us worriers to *turn off* parts of our brains, and eliminate stress, but we can make the effort. Exercise, meditation, aggressively tackling looming life choices or issues, a closer spiritual presence in our lives, whatever it takes to minimize stress levels, it is worth making the effort.

ALLOW YOUR MIND TO RELAX OCCASSIONALLY, FIND YOUR GO TO PLACE; THROUGH EXERCISE OR MEDITATION / PRAYING, CURLING UP WITH A GOOD BOOK OR A HOT BATH, A WALK IN WOODS OR

GAZING AT THE NIGHT SKY, WHATEVER BRINGS YOUR MIND TO THAT MOMENT OF PEACE, FIND IT AND DON'T FORGET TO GO THERE SOMETIMES.

While we may or may not have much success changing our thought patterns, and processes, we do have many choices and options available that help us take care of our physical bodies. This helps keep our bodies strong, and in optimum condition to fight in the event of a severe illness or at the onset of disease.

MAKING THE EFFORT TO MAINTAIN A HEALTHY BODY THROUGH PROPER NUTRITION, REST AND EXERCISE IS BASIC COMMON SENSE AND A WISE CHOICE.

So is there a formula, a recipe to follow that would help determine who is likely to develop cancer and who is not? Is anyone really any safer than anyone else? Look all around us; everywhere we turn we face new health threats.

THERE HAVE BEEN GENETICALLY MODIFIED FOODS STOCKED ON THE GROCERY SHELVES FOR OUR CONSUMPTION SINCE EARLY ON IN THE 1990'S.

Did you know that since it was determined through clinical studies that we as Americans do not eat enough food products containing omega 3 that it was considered a great scientific advancement that we now have tomato plants with fish genes genetically spliced in? Crops like corn and wheat, major staple products, have pesticide and herbicide components built right in at the genetic DNA level. This was intended to reduce the use of chemical pesticide and herbicide applications in agricultural practices. This was because they were concerned these chemicals would, and did, build up to toxic levels in the soil. Instead of applying pesticides to the plant as it grew, they began incorporating these properties into the plant itself. You may have heard mention of GM plants in association with conversation regarding dwindling bee and monarch butterfly populations?

TODAY ORGANIC PRODUCTS HAVE BECOME VERY POPULAR, BUT DID YOU KNOW THAT GM CROPS CAN BE LABELED AS ORGANIC?

This is because the organic certification process covers what is *added* to the soil *during* the growth phases of the plant. It does not include properties that are integral components, part of the plant, from within the seed itself.

Everyone should make a point of learning the basic coding system used to translate the mysterious PLU codes that are found on all fresh fruit, vegetables and bulk produce items such as nuts and herbs. Unless it is from a name brand, in which case they are not required to have an established PLU under IFPS.

You know that little number that is there to help the stores keep track of inventory and register prices within the computer system? That same little number can tell you whether or not the produce you are paying to eat is really what you think it is. These codes were established fairly recently and are controlled by the **INTERNATIONAL FEDERATION FOR PRODUCE STANDARDS** (IFPS). Since it is a fairly new system it is subject to change, for that reason I would recommend a simple internet search to determine information regarding the codes that are currently in effect.

HUMAN GROWTH HORMONES ARE PREVALENT IN MANY FOODS WE CONSUME, FROM MILK IN THE EARLY 1990'S AND DAIRY PRODUCTS TO ALL MANNER BEEF AND POULTRY MEATS AND PRODUCTS AND BY PRODUCTS.

There have been a number of studies that indicate that HgH may have an association in the rise in diabetes incidents.

MULTIPLE REPORTS FOUND THAT LARGE DOSES OF HGH CAUSED A MARKED INSULIN RESISTANCE INCREASE IN SOME INDIVIDUALS, WHICH WOULD TRANSLATE TO AN INCREASE IN BLOOD GLUCOSE LEVELS FOR DIABETICS.

It cannot actually be proven at this time that HgH is a direct cause of developing diabetes. Multiple studies and sources do provide supporting evidence though that exhibit there does appear to be a direct correlation, a definite affect and/or interaction that occurs between HgH and our bodies sugar processing abilities.

We have watched over the past two decades as America's economy became more and more pharmaceutically driven. We are the "take a pill generation", a topic so deep, it is a standalone issue. It has become quite common knowledge that many pharmaceutical by-products, prescription medications and poorly managed sanitary and manufacturing waste products have seriously polluted our fresh water drinking supplies.

Whether you buy bottled or not, you still throw the dice that one source is in reality any better than the other. If it is not bad enough that the food and water that is needed by every living thing for survival has become questionable, there are also major air quality issues.

This is due to *known* human contributions like the cars we all drive, rocket ships, air travel, manufacturing facilities and power production plants for example, and *unknown* and questionable contributions, such as chemtrailing operations by aircraft. These operations can range from chemical pesticide applications and fertilizing, to weather modification efforts and who knows what else. It has only recently become common knowledge to those inquisitive enough to investigate the topic that chemtrailing is no longer a *conspiracy theorist* topic only. There is a clear differentiation to be made between *contrails*, which are normal aircraft exhaust with visibility and color dependent upon altitude, temperature and weather conditions at the time and *Chemtrails*, which are chemicals intentionally dispensed and dispersed in flight via a variety of systems installed in a wide range of aircraft models, from single engine to large Jets, over a large area. You can now even find career opportunities with weather modification companies. Indeed some of the problems with the air, food and water conditions discussed seem so unbelievable and have such a science fiction, end of the world sound to them it is a wonder cancer rates are not even higher.

The study of illnesses, such as cancer rates, autism, diabetes and arthritis just to name a few is another stand alone topic that begs deeper investigation. One may think it would be very easy to examine these rates using the statistics composed for this very purpose and available through sources such as the government CDC website. What I have found though is the CDC files available to the general public begin with 1999. Since most of these controversial food products and chemical applications began in the 1990's other sources would definitely be needed. How can you compare autism or cancer rates prior to GM food introductions versus ten years post public introduction for example if you are not able to access statistics from the years prior to the introduction?

These topics and others of great interest and importance are covered in much greater depth in the soon to be released *Everything You Ever Wanted to Know About... That Mainstream Media, Members of Congress and the Mega Corporations Were Afraid Someday You Would Ask*, WHAT TO EXPECT WHEN YOU'RE EXPECTING CANCER is about being a survivor.

You may accept all, only a portion or none of the concerns regarding our food sources or air and water quality issues as discussed to be factual, but truthfully? Whether you worry about if you will get cancer or not, chances are that at some time, to some degree, you have been exposed to one form of carcinogen or another in the course of your life while innocently going about your daily activities. Like it or not these unknown variables must be included as part of the ingredients in any formula created that is trying to determine the recipe for who is most likely to develop cancer.

As if food, air and water issues are not disconcerting enough, we are still not done with the almost unlimited combination of variables that affect efforts to create this formula to accurately categorize who may be more prone to developing cancer and who is not. The mixing bowl requires the addition of two very important missing ingredients that still need to be added to the impartial blender blades of chance.

One of these missing elements is our own hereditary DNA passed down through our personal family trees. These are inherent genetic qualities directly passed on to you by your mother and father, and your ancestors. When we are born we all have two copies of each gene. We all get one set from each individual parent. Hereditary cancers can occur if there is a change or mutation to a damage-controlling gene in one of these copies. These are the genes which normally help protect our bodies against development of radical abnormal cancer cells. In almost all instances these are genetic changes that were passed on from either the mother or father's side of the family.

THERE IS A 50% POSSIBILITY THAT THE PARENT WITH THE DEFECTIVE GENE WILL PASS THE MUTATION OR DAMAGE ALONG TO THEIR CHILD.

People at high risk for cancer due to an inherited mutation are said to have genetic susceptibility. Having an identified genetic mutation does not mean that you will definitely develop cancer though. It may indicate you are more prone though. For example Squamous cell carcinoma is the type of lung cancer most strongly linked to family history. If you have a family history of Squamous cell carcinoma lung cancer, whether you smoke or not, your gender, which relative had lung cancer, can all affect the odds of whether or not *you* will develop lung cancer. Some examples of cancers most commonly associated with the high risk genetic susceptibility category include breast and ovarian cancer, bladder, and colon cancers, as well as Multiple Endocrine Neoplasia II, which can involve the thyroid, adrenal, Parathyroid glands. These are factors that can affect your chances of developing cancer that are not chosen. An individual does not have control over inherited variables, but there are other contributing factors, *ingredients*, that we very much do have control over.

Into this formula we have thus far, a combination of everyday exposures and inherited traits, we must now slowly fold in all of the bad habits that we have indulged in over the course of our lifetimes. Gently stirring in to the batter as we go a slew of impurities, representing the life choices we have made. These life choices, the habits and indulgences that need to be added for most of us will be many. They may have been choices as innocent as choosing a poor sugar substitute in a well intended effort to maintain a healthy weight; or a purely bad, conscious choice such as smoking. Especially since the new FSC Fire Safe Compliant Cigarettes were released and it was made law that all cigarettes sold comply. These FSC cigarettes have added a whole new class of chemicals to the smoke inhaled, not only for the smoker's lungs and thereby the blood stream, but unfortunately this is true for the victims of second hand smoke fumes as well.

We pour and spoon the bad stuff into the mixing bowl in accordance with how we have moved through life, in various measures, in dashes and pinches. Besides the big obvious bad life choice of smoking, there is also excessive drinking and/or drug addictions. Either or both of which can negatively impact many other bodily functions related to our bodies' purification and filtration abilities. These adverse effects may become evident by partial to complete failure of any number of bodily functions, from the kidneys and liver, to nutritional absorption and bowel movements. If the body is not able to clear a particular waste product, either in the form of urine, sweat, or fecal movements, where does it go? The body must store it somewhere. Many feel the most common place is within fat cells. If this is true then not only are the big bad obvious life choices like smoking, drinking and drug abuse major contributors to the game of chance known as who can get cancer, but some of the more innocent life choices as well, such as what we eat, or how much we exercise. In this age of automation and instant gratification lack of exercise is often coupled with poor diet choices that involve unregulated consumption of sweets and/or highly processed foods, and GM foods that perhaps are not processed the same. I feel that because of this we have seen the obesity rates increase across the board, regardless of age, income or race. So if fat cells are storage cells, is it possible that they are environmentally *friendly* to cancer cells? Either in a nurturing, breeding ground sense of the word, or perhaps as a source of easily accessible fuel for radical fast multiplying cells? If this is so, then being overweight may be more hazardous to your health than previously thought.

These are just a few personal choices from a long list that is seemingly endless. Today, even if you do eat well and stay active outdoors, simpler choices, such as failure to use proper sunscreen protection can increase your risks.

When we have added all of our personal life choices to our existing mix of food, water and environmental impurities, and our own hereditary DNA risks, most of us will realize that the dish is quite toxic. Can we really determine or predict with any accuracy who can or will get cancer and who will not? I do not think so.

ALL, OR A COMBINATION OF ANY OF A COUNTLESS NUMBER OF FACTORS COULD CONSPIRE TO WORK AGAINST US, COULD MAKE US BECOME POTENTIAL CANCER SURVIVORS.

In my case I have always pretty much considered myself indestructible. I had a pre-formed picture of myself someday growing old and doling out sound advice to the whippersnappers from a rocking chair, with nice plumpy cushions for my bony butt and back, on the front porch. I'm not a heavy drinker, although in my youth I did pass through a brief "party" phase, I am not big on processed foods and high sugar content treats, and to the best of my knowledge there was no history of cancer within the biological family tree. All good things going for me by today's standards you could say. I was into amateur body building and considered quite fit, trim and active; but I was a smoker.

It was actually within three months of the FSC Fire Safe Compliant cigarettes "officially" hitting the stores that I became really sick. I believe the release was in April; it was in June that I again made myself go to the doctor. In late August, after I had lost my voice completely for over two weeks I was referred to an Ear Nose Throat Specialist. I was diagnosed with stage IVB throat cancer on my birthday October 13th. I will add that smoking cigarettes has not been my only risk factor. I have also spent most of my adult life as a painting contractor in the construction industry. This involved multiple risk factors ranging from using spray painting systems and working around finely misted airborne paint products; to possibly coming in contact with substances such as asbestos and lead paints through sanding and heat applications during remodels and restorations, which I specialized in.

There are a number of professions that result in daily exposure to known carcinogens that often we just never really think about, it's just part of the job. Repeat exposure creates a higher risk. That was why from the 1980's we saw all the gas stations going self serve. It wasn't so bad for you to gas up your car once or twice a week, but it wasn't healthy for the poor gas jockey's pumping, sometimes hundreds of tanks a day, day after day. So what the gas manufacturers did was a move similar to the liquor industry. When activist sought to have hard liquor commercials banned from television air time, the industry removed them 'voluntarily'. We saw in the early 1990's new laws were discussed, but nothing passed to limit employee hours of exposure. Then almost overnight self serve gasoline stations became the rage. Since 2002 we are seeing the trends go the other way again, with some states even passing laws that you had to be a qualified attendant to be allowed to pump gas.

One thing I do know, we can make the right choices to *decrease* our risks of developing cancer of one type or another, but we cannot *eliminate* them.

Quite frankly, between the oil disaster in the Gulf of the United States, and the even more recent nuclear disaster in Japan, can ANY of us say with any certainty at all that we will not develop cancer? Or that we have not thought about the possibility?

I would recommend if you are undiagnosed at this time, and already eat a healthy diet, and you are making conscious, well informed choices towards maintaining your health, know the early warning signs to look for, just keep up the good work and let go of the worries. Do not let fear and uncertainty of the unknowns in your future rob you of happiness while living your life and enjoying the precious moments.

IN ANSWER TO THE QUESTION WHO GETS CANCER AND WHO DOES NOT? THERE IS NO SATISFACTORY ANSWER. AS SCARY AS THE THOUGHT IS, AS MUCH AS WE WOULD LIKE TO THINK NOT, THE FACT IS THAT ANYONE COULD DEVELOP CANCER. PERHAPS THE MORE IMPORTANT QUESTION SHOULD BE WHO SURVIVES CANCER, AND WHY?

3 LEARN TO LISTEN TO OURSELVES

Learning to Listen to Ourselves is about watching for or being aware of some of the much more subtle clues our body and our minds may use to communicate that something is wrong… even if at every doctor's appointment you have been told everything is normal. If it is true that there is no way to accurately predict who may get cancer and it is a fact that it is possible for anyone to develop cancer, whether due to hereditary factors or through environmental and/or lifestyle triggers as previously discussed, then what *can* an individual do to protect themselves? Learn to Listen to Your Body.

One of the major problems in dealing with cancer today is that many cancers are silent. Cancers may be symptom free, or may produce only vague, sometimes come and go symptoms. This is especially true in the early to mid-stage progression of the disease. It is because of this lack of definitive symptoms that many cancers are unfortunately not detected until they have progressed quite far. This is very unfortunate, because there are a number of cancers that respond quite well to early intervention treatments. I was diagnosed at a very advanced Stage IV B, which is only one letter grade from Stage IVC. Stage IVC disease is considered to be at a stage that it is incurable or terminal. In general, for all but the most deadly types of cancers, the earlier a diagnosis is made and treatment is begun, the more favorable the patient's prognosis and outcome will be.

EARLY DETECTION OF CANCER IS YOUR BEST DEFENSE AGAINST CANCER.

So if discovering cancer early is so crucial to surviving, to completing a successful treatment regimen, how can we better the odds of detecting it? Are there specific symptoms to watch for that should raise a red flag? When should you call the doctor?

Getting to know yourself and your body better will help you develop an awareness of even small changes in *your* body's functions, appearances and sometimes even your thought processes. This is why I like to say, no one knows your body better than you. Only you are going to be aware of very subtle changes, physically as well as mentally, that your body uses to communicate.

WHEN YOUR BODY SAYS HOUSTON WE HAVE A PROBLEM, IT IS WISE TO PAY ATTENTION TO THE CLUES.

Earlier in the year that I was diagnosed with Squamous cell carcinoma of the supraglottis as well as my larynx, I did notice a number of oddities. Upon looking back in retrospect I think these were subtle warning signs. To be honest I refer to them as subtle, but in reality I think my body was screaming out to me with the only voice it had, and I failed to listen.

For example, even though I had been experiencing and ignoring fatigue at the time, I went on a major cleaning binge. This was similar to what you may have heard described as *nesting syndrome,* associated with new expectant mothers. I was cleaning closets, file cabinets, painting rooms. I could not stop myself. It was like I was driven. Almost like I *knew* that soon my home would be welcoming a flood of guests on a long rotating basis, and that I knew I would not be able to get the house ready, unless I did it then.

I also experienced a family photo organizing obsession. I mean I went through photo albums, and shoeboxes, hundreds and hundreds of photos, and uploaded the chosen ones on to my social network utility. I worried that if anything happened to me where would all of these old photographs end up? I wanted all four of my children to be able to print out their own family photo albums. It was our history. I worried that if I did not get these photos organized and uploaded to my social utility page that many of them would be lost forever... if anything happened to me. My husband was quite frustrated with me at the time; after all I could not play the cancer card for sympathy at that point. I had piles of photos and frames laid about in three different rooms of our house for over two weeks. Yes, you read correctly I said frames. This obsession included taking down framed photos from off of the walls for scanning.

The words *obsessed* and *driven* in regards to my cleaning binge, and photo preservation activities are strong words, and I am not using them lightly. This was out of the ordinary behavior that was accompanied by a suppressed sense of desperation, a feeling of time running out.

I say again it is important to know yourself. For some individuals these obsessive behaviors may be an unfortunate everyday part of their lives that they have learned or must learn to live with. There are also many people prone to what are known as anxiety attacks.

ONLY *YOU* WILL RECOGNIZE WHAT IS YOUR NORMAL STATE OF MIND.

I did recognize my behavior as weird for me, but at the time did not know why it was happening. I mean when the house was ready top to bottom, my obsessive need to clean vanished. When I reached a point that I was satisfied all of the important old family related photos would be easily accessible to all of my children, everything else went back into photo albums, boxes and storage, and I was done.

Choosing to tackle either of these chores may be considered *normal* for some, including myself. We all need to top to bottom the house occasionally, spring cleaning you know? So the urge to complete a thorough cleaning was *nothing new*. Today many young people, in this age of digital media, are not even accustomed to seeing old black and white photographs that you actually hold in your hand. Computers have made photograph storage and cataloging very convenient. Those in the baby boomer age group, as I am, and others who are older, would probably admit that having urges and good intentions to organize our photograph collections would be *nothing new*. For me it was not *what* I wanted to accomplish that was *new*, it was the *driving / obsessive* need that had pushed me to complete those tasks, ASAP that was.

I used the words obsessed and driven because while I worked at accomplishing these tasks I found that I was functioning under the overpowering sense that there was a strictly established and enforceable timeline allowed that I was supposed to accomplish the projects within. In my humble opinion I think that these particular *clues* were based upon a pre-existing close spiritual relationship. It would be impossible to attempt a truly detailed explanation in regards to sharing my own personal "religious" beliefs as you will no doubt learn by the end of this small book, let us just say they include ideals that some may find peculiar. I will delve a little deeper into this relationship within these pages but for the moment, at this point and time, let it suffice to say that Yes I do believe there is definitely a Higher Power, just not in the accepted over organized strictly regulated sense of "religion". When the big Man tells you to do something, you know it, and you do it, it's as simple as that.

There have been numerous papers written that indicate many individuals either prior to death, or during a particularly life threatening health crisis or accident, have experienced similar, what I call communications or messages of a spiritual nature. Often this is perceived as an impending sense of doom; a premonition of approaching death, or mortality, a glimpse into the beyond. In many cases this sense of impending mortality occurs in the complete absence of a recognized or diagnosed imminent threat.

There has been a great deal of research regarding this particular aspect of religion and spiritual communication, and a number of respected well written manuscripts have been published. One such book that I found to be extremely well researched and written, in my opinion founded upon credible experiences, was written by a Dr. Allan Hamilton. The doctor's book, called *The Scalpel and the Soul* (2008), was based upon his experiences with patients that spanned a course of three decades during his career as a Harvard-educated brain surgeon. Doctor Hamilton discusses numerous experiences involving this phenomenon.

My Father experienced one of these strong premonitions, just prior to his unexpected death. My Dad (I was adopted, but in my heart and mind, and theirs the Sweet family was my family) was a Veteran of the Korean War, and he did have existing health concerns that we were all aware of. None of which we thought placed him at immediate risk though. He was under a doctor's care through the Veterans administration, and was very responsible about taking his medications. I lived over a thousand miles from my parents at this time. I had four brothers, and over the years in between periods of boot camp, living on base, and deployments, at least one always maintained homes in Upstate New York at all times, close to Mom and Dad. At this time, years before my diagnosis, our brother Dean lived right across the road. One day, out of the blue, just over a year after Mom passed away, Dad decided that Mom's engagement ring had to be mailed to me; That Very Day. My brother's wife called me, because he was really raising a ruckus over this. He had begun insisting early in the morning, and was persistent into the afternoon. The ring had to be mailed to me, that day. They said he was very agitated, even threatening to attempt to walk to the post office himself. It was winter. When they finally did relent, and told him they would go, they said he calmed down somewhat, but insisted he would want to see a receipt from the post office when they returned home. It was only after he had that receipt in hand that they said he settled down, and seemed happy. My Father passed away before the ring arrived in Georgia. He died in his sleep that night. My brother Dean said when he found him in the morning he was laying on his left side, with his head in the crook of arm, looking completely at peace, as though sleeping. Dad had suffered a massive stroke.

Of course I cannot say for sure whether the ring would have come to me without Dad's intervention. First of all none of us had even been aware of where the ring was. I had actually thought it was with Mom. Also, my brother's do love me, but I was adopted after all, and our youngest brother was leaning towards getting married at the time. There were also four granddaughters bearing the Sweet family name. When I went up for the funeral, a sad but *"Sweet"* Sweet family reunion would we have found the ring while I was there, and would it have come back home with me? I do not know. We did not even know until the funeral service, which was attended by a Veterans Military representative who presented us with a flag, that Dad was awarded 3 bronze stars during his military service. He never told us. It was when we went back to his home after the service, that the topic of his little lock box came up. It was where he had retrieved Mom's ring from just a few days earlier. There in the box, along with some small black and white wallet size photos of the ship he sailed off to war on, and a few photos of fellow soldiers, with names we'll never know, a few old coins, and two gold teeth, and a baby picture of me (I was adopted at age six), we found the three bronze stars. Dad was a good man, not prone to a lot of emotional discussion, and very humble. Did he truly have a premonition of death? I think he did. More than that, I think he had a spiritual communication. It was not just because Dad *wanted* me to have the ring, but because somehow he knew I would *need* it in my future.

EVERYTHING HAPPENS FOR A REASON.

To some people that little ring may have been considered very nondescript and of little value, but for me it signified so much more. The letter Dad sent with the ring was brief, but he had said he wanted me to have the ring because "I would need it". For a couple of years I kept the ring in a special place, afraid that if I wore it I would lose it, *before I needed it*. When I was diagnosed, I began wearing the ring because I knew the time was right. I put it on my pinky, the only finger it would fit. God Bless her, Mom's hands were very tiny and petite. For me that little ring became a constant source of comfort and strength, a powerful symbol of family, Mom and Dad, and love. It reminded me every day that I was not alone, Mom and Dad encouraged me onward through the grueling treatment regime that lasted for over two months. To me that ring is priceless, and to this day I thank the Higher Power for prompting Dad to be so insistent that day. One thing I have not mentioned… my Mom died from throat cancer.

SO, while mental state of mind *messages* or warning signs may be more difficult to recognize for what they are at the time they are happening, it is possible that they may be considered as a symptom, an indication that something is wrong. I am sure many people, like I did, may miss understanding and recognizing these obsessive driving urges to accomplish tasks, until after the facts unfold, as the spiritual message they really were.

AN OBSESSIVE DRIVING NEED TO ACCOMPLISH SPECIFIC TASKS MAY TRULY BE A PREMONITION OR WARNING OF THE PRESENCE OF AN UNKNOWN ILLNESS.

Besides spiritual communications that I feel occur within the brain, our bodies have a number of other ways to communicate distress or needs to us that sometimes we tend to over look.

Very early on I had found myself experiencing particular food cravings. I am talking desires for certain foods that if you took all of the cravings experienced in the course of all four of my pregnancies, combined, they could not hold a candle to my odd desires. These yearnings were so incredibly strong, and very specific. If I did not get the item I wanted, at the time I wanted it, I experienced mood changes that were not pretty. Cover your ears and excuse my French but, quite frankly, I became a bitch.

I BELIEVE FOOD CRAVINGS MAY BE ONE OF THE MORE SUBTLE OF MESSAGES THAT COME FROM YOUR INNER BODY AS A WAY OF SIGNALING US THERE IS A PROBLEM.

I also wondered if men had experienced similar food cravings prior to or early on in their cancer diagnosis, so I set out to ask questions. Surprisingly I found during the long course of my treatment, through conversations with the male population of my compatriots at The Winship Cancer Center, that many of them had also experienced food cravings prior to diagnosis. The desires included a broad range of food items from a wide variety of vegetables and fruits, to specific types of chocolates. We all shared welcome light hearted laughter over the idea of men experiencing the pregnancy like symptoms of mood swings and food cravings.

For me the strongest and longest lasting food craving, which persisted until I could no longer swallow anything but thick liquids and smooth mush, was nuts. I went nuts for nuts, and could not get enough them. At first it was almost any kind of nut, but over the course of time this urge had refined itself to pistachios and almonds. Asparagus was another food item I found myself wanting abnormally. I mean don't get me wrong, I liked nuts and asparagus, but this was more like a *Need*. I was eating nuts every day, and asparagus 3-5 times a week. I preferred fresh asparagus, with butter and lots of pepper, fresh ground pepper mélange, but I would eat the canned asparagus in a pinch. You will no doubt find this somewhat gross, but I kept cans of tips and spears in the cabinets, and sometimes I would open one up and eat them cold right out of the can. I mean seriously, it even sounds gross to me now too, but I was doing it then.

IT IS A NORMAL PROCESS FOR THE BODY TO CRAVE SOMETHING IT LACKS. SOME CRAVINGS UPON INVESTIGATION AND DISCUSSION WITH YOUR PRIMARY DOCTOR AND ROUTINE BLOOD TEST COULD REVEAL A SIMPLE VITAMIN OR MINERAL DEFICIENCY. THIS HAPPENS ALL THE TIME, AND IS QUITE NATURAL, BUT CRAVINGS SHOULD BE INVESTIGATED.

In the case of cancer though I think this craving for certain foods is a bit more complex. Instead of being a reaction to an existing deficiency these cravings may be more about building up defenses against a future deficiency. The body is doing more than requesting additional *nutrition*; I think it is requesting more *ammunition*. It did not occur to me until I was already scheduled for my biopsy to use a search engine and ask what health conditions a few of these cravings were good for. Asparagus and almonds for example are repeatedly cited in numerous articles and studies as having a broad spectrum of cancer prevention, slowing, and / or healing properties. Lately even dark chocolate has switched sides and has been noted in moderation as one of the good guys now. Either way intense, specific food cravings at the very least do deserve some investigation to determine any underlying cause.

Aside from messages such as premonitions that we can say are mental signs, and food cravings sent out by our bodies that can be considered inner physical signs, there are of course many more common, expected and feared cancer symptoms as well. These are outer physical symptoms.

Cancer symptoms and early warning signs as we know can differ greatly from one individual to the next. This happens not only because of an individual's current physical health at the onset of disease, but because of many other variables. There are currently in excess of 200 hundred different types and forms of cancer, and we have 60 different organs in our bodies, any one or more in which cancer may develop. It is even possible to have more than one type of cancer at the same time. So it is quite easy to understand why symptoms vary so greatly. Many people are aware of the more common warning signs of cancer, but they are worth reviewing.

Fatigue is one of those very vague symptoms that may come and go, making it very difficult to attribute a cause to. Sometimes we think well it was just a really busy week, or maybe I'm coming down with a bug, or I've overdone it. Fatigue is probably one the most misdiagnosed symptoms in the world. It is also one of the ailments most likely to be quickly and incorrectly treated with anti-depressant medications.

An unexplained and unintentional weight loss is another symptom that often accompanies fatigue. Substantial drops in an otherwise steady weight could be indicative of serious health problems. During the period that I was experiencing elevated calcium and muscle enzyme levels I did lose ten pounds, but then the weight loss stabilized for well over eight months. This stabilization seems to have coincided with the changes I had experienced in my eating habits.

The appearance of any new moles, or changes that occur to existing moles resulting in irregular raised borders, or dark splotchy color variations, should be investigated. Non-melanoma skin cancer has become the most diagnosed form of cancer. Any skin changes for that matter, for example a sore that won't heal, an orange peel appearance to areas of skin or small lumps found just below the surface, should not immediately serve to bring on a panic attack, but they definitely warrant a trip to the doctor's office. Occasionally, standing in front of a mirror and making a visual body check is a good idea as well. At the same time you can lightly explore areas with your fingertips, pressing lightly, to search for any hidden lumps or lymph nodes, being especially attentive to areas of soft mass, such as the breast and stomach. Women in particular, paying special attention to breast health, besides lumps, should also take note of any itching, redness or changes to the areola area. Women should also know their menstruation cycle. Unusual discharge, bleeding between menstrual cycles, and heavy periods should really make you consider a consultation with a good doctor. Studies have indicated that for women worldwide the average percentage over the course of their lifetimes that will develop ovarian cancer is at 1 in 70. Within the U.S. these figures are even more alarming, coming in at 1 in 55. That means that almost half of the women's population within the United States is at risk of developing ovarian cancer.

IF IN THE COURSE OF HOME EXAMINATIONS YOU DO DISCOVER SOMETHING OUT OF THE NORM, DO NOT PANIC; OFTEN LUMPS AND SKIN CHANGES, EVEN WHEN COMBINED WITH UNEXPLAINED PERIODS OF FATIGUE OR WEIGHT LOSS ARE NOT A RESULT OF CANCER, BUT ASSOCIATED WITH OTHER BENIGN LESS OMINOUS BODILY PROCESSES.

There are also a number of other symptoms that should really catch your attention. This would include for example any rectal bleeding or blood in stools that cannot be attributed to hemorrhoids, or even changes in your regular bowel habits. A persistent cough, hoarseness, or difficulty swallowing, enlarged lymph nodes, especially in the neck, or a sore throat or neck pain that last more than two weeks should be investigated. Remember I walked around with cancer growing in my throat for a very long time, and it was not until I lost my voice, for two full weeks, that I was sent to an ENT.

Again I say, know your body, and listen to it when it speaks to you. Any of these symptoms discussed should be considered as warning signs, not to be ignored. For that matter *any* persistent symptom that lasts a month or more without resolution should be a reason to visit your physician.

There are a number of blood tests available that are utilized to indicate the presence of very specific types of cancer. For example it has been found that CA 15.3 values are very often elevated in patients with breast cancer. CA125 may be used as a tumor marker for women suspected to have cancers of the reproductive system that may include the uterus, fallopian tubes and ovaries. There are even new blood tests that are able to screen for markers that may indicate the presence of 13 different types of cancers all at once. Screening for active Epstein Bar virus (EBV) can also be used as an indicative cancer marker for nasopharyngeal cancer. These are only a few examples of blood tests that may be used to screen for cancer markers. So if there are so many simple blood tests available that can screen for cancer why can't we all just get a bunch of blood tests you ask?

The problem with just randomly screening for cancer is that like symptoms the markers may be caused by a number of other issues besides cancer. For example a common cancer marker known as Carcinoembryonic antigen (CEA), which is associated with digestive tract cancers of the colon, as well as Medullary thyroid cancer (MTC) may show as a false positive, because these levels may be elevated by treatable non cancerous digestive disorders as well. The CA125 tests, as well as the more advanced CA125-II, which is used as an ovarian cancer screen may be elevated during normal bodily functions, such as menstruation, or pregnancy. Non cancerous ovarian cysts, and active diseases and conditions, such as pericarditis, hepatitis, or peritonitis, (an infection of the lining of the abdomen), can result in elevations or false positives as a cancer screening tool. The CA125 tests could even show elevated markers in a low percentage of 100% healthy individuals. So in other words, I am not saying that these are not diagnostic tests we should count on, only that I would not request them unless there were symptoms specific to a cancer concern, or if there is a known hereditary risk factor.

THERE ARE MANY BLOOD TESTS AVAILABLE THAT ARE USED TO DETECT ELEVATED CANCER MARKERS, BUT IT IS IMPORTANT TO REMEMBER THAT FOR EACH OF THESE

TESTS THERE ARE A NUMBER OF BENIGN, NON CANCEROUS CONDITIONS THAT MAY CAUSE FALSE POSITIVES, AND UNNECESSARY FEAR.

The Epstein Barr testing I found especially interesting and surprising to learn about, because I myself had elevated EBV results. This was many, many years before my diagnosis or any symptoms. Yes, I said years. I found it absolutely mind boggling when I learned that. Imagine over six years passed since that blood test that was considered *interesting* to the doctor, but *inconsequential*. I was told that everyone had dormant EBV markers in their blood. Mine was only interesting because at that time they were active. I still had a high school age teenager at home back then though, and the doctor suspected a simple active infection was present and prescribed an antibiotic. The elevations were put off as possible exposure to mononucleosis, which would have totally explained the presence of the active EPV in the blood work. Scary thought though isn't it? Cancer was growing inside of me for possibly 7 years plus or minus, and I did not know. No wonder it had reached the point of stage IV B.

There are a number of steps we will take as we walk through the closing stages of the period of our *Life Before Cancer*. If you have suffered from any, or many of symptoms discussed that are consistent with a specific cancer type you have hopefully been working in close contact with your physician. If your doctor has run corresponding blood tests that resulted in elevated markers indicating the presence of a suspected cancer type, you have most likely already been scheduled for further testing. CT scans or MRI images of the area or organ thought to be affected have most likely been completed by now. This part of your journey is almost complete now.

Your final steps in that old life will most likely lead to the operating room to obtain tissue samples. This surgery is called a biopsy, and it is done to determine if the abnormal cells are malignant or benign. If the cells are malignant then type of specific cancer cells present are usually identified at this time as well. The doctor will also visually inspect the affected area and/or organs. In some cases during this surgery if it is possible or recommended some tumors are surgically removed at this time, or they may only be partially removed to relieve pressure on adjoining structures. It will be based on this visualization and viewing the CT, PET scans and/or MRI images if cancer is present that your cancer will be *staged*. When you awaken it will be time to take your first steps into a new world filled with many unknowns ahead of you. The world known as Life With Cancer.

May your footfalls be firm and steady, your gaze to the future and your attitude positive.

SECTION II: LIFE WITH CANCER

4 DIAGNOSIS: A STATE OF MIND

So you have been diagnosed with cancer. Does it really matter where it is? Or what type? It's scary. Would it be any less fear inspiring to hear that the abnormally growing radical cells that have invaded were in one body part or another? I do not think so, unless perhaps you have expertise within the medical profession. In which case you may be educated enough to rapidly access the almost innumerable variables and roughly estimate based on cancer type, location and stage what the average chances would be for successful treatment to the point of complete cure. The average person diagnosed with cancer does not have this wealth of information immediately at hand, although many will go online to research and view available statistics and information. *Diagnosis: A State of Mind* is about the beginning of living life During Cancer, and about not short changing the chances of survival for yourself or your loved one based on what you may read in reports and statistics about seemingly similar cases.

I BELIEVE IF WE SET TOO MUCH STORE, BASE OUR OWN CHANCES OF SURVIVAL ON THE NUMBERS PREDICTED BY SCIENCE AND RESEARCH STATISTICS SOME MAY SHORT CHANGE THEMSELVES, DOUBTING SURVIVAL FROM THE START.

Luckily prior to diagnosis we have most likely not read too many of these depressing and deceptive, coldly calculating, impersonal papers that are intended to estimate cancer survival statistics. What do I mean many of the statistics are depressing? What do I mean deceptive?

They are depressing because first of all you will find almost every single one of these studies are presented and projected based upon five year survival rates. So right off the bat they *imply* a feeling of, or lead one to believe that, five years is an accepted *normal* or *average* outlook for life expectancy after a cancer diagnosis. I have no idea why the majority of studies available have chosen this five year format, but remember this:

YOU DO NOT HAVE A FIVE YEAR EXPIRATION DATE AFTER A CANCER DIAGNOSIS; THERE ARE MANY PEOPLE WHO HAVE SURVIVED FOR DECADES, LONG AFTER TREATMENT, FOR A GREAT NUMBER OF CANCER TYPES.

Myths and misunderstandings like this are one of the reasons I recommend if you, or a loved one has been diagnosed with cancer, as discussed in *Going The Distance*, join a reputable, well established support group, as soon as possible. The internet offers many, and I discuss two of the very best. Within these forums you will be able to find not only answers to your questions, friendship and support, but many long term survivors as well. These are the alumni graduates from the School of Hard Knocks, the cancer survivors, and they are one of the greatest sources for information and inspiration available. You will be able to judge for yourself, and thereby be assured, that yes there are many people who actually do go on to enjoy quite full lives beyond cancer. You will find for yourself that there are many people, not numbers, but *people*, who have survived cancer well beyond five years. These are individuals who not only reached the point and time in treatment that the light at the end of the tunnel began to shine bright enough to dispel the cloying reach of the dark shadow cast by cancer; but people who have put on their sunglasses and continued their journey forward into bright sunshine, *far* beyond the five year survival rates that are depicted in cancer survival statistics.

As if predictions were not depressing or deceptive enough, just because they are based upon a five year outlook, there is another reason I say they are flawed.

I CONTEND THAT SINCE THESE PREDICTIONS ARE BASED UPON EQUATIONS THAT REQUIRE THE INPUT OF SPECIFIC NUMERICAL DATA TO ARRIVE AT THEIR CONCLUSIONS, THE STATISTICS CANNOT POSSIBLY BE CONSIDERED ACCURATE BECAUSE THEY DO NOT HAVE ALL THE NUMBERS NECESSARY.

Any formula intended to predict outcomes, based upon observation and experimentation, comparing data sets assembled over a course of time, will require the assignment of an established error margin, which is based upon variables. The variables are the missing numbers required to accurately complete the equation. So where exactly are these missing variables to be found, and what makes their numerical values so difficult to determine? It is the human factor.

I personally disagree with lumping people together and *fitting* them into categories, but, for the purpose of this discussion, let's say we had to *try*. I have observed and recognized in the course of my personal cancer experience that there seems to be three distinct types of cancer patients.

A) There are a percentage of individuals in the survival statistic equations that *want* or *expect* to survive. These are those who besides making a conscious decision to fight, somehow *know* they *could* win. Whether through education or guidance from an *inner* source, these will make preparations, do all the *right* things, and stay strong. This in turn enables them to meet, and beat, the demanding and exhausting cancer treatment regime'.

B) There is another distinct group that also consists of individuals who *want* to survive, may even *expect* to survive. Within this group though, for a number of reasons we find some that do not survive the treatments. This is an important distinction to understand. What I am saying is that they did not succumb to the cancer, but, to the treatment. Cancer treatments, whether you have radiation, chemotherapy, or a combination of both, as I did, are very hard on the body, and considered quite toxic.

I feel the reason some may weaken, and succumb to the treatments is initiated by a number of factors. For example high stress levels that can be brought on by concerns such as scheduling and travel issues, lack of support, failing to stick to treatment schedule, financial difficulties, and many may also include problems such as pre-existing health conditions, or lifestyle habits that they were unable to conquer or control such as drugs or alcohol. Any, or a combination of these obstacles, many of which are avoidable to an extent, could weaken an individual to the verge of succumbing to the very treatments intended to save them.

C) Lastly is our third group. These are the individuals who do not *expect* to survive, and who are comfortable and at peace with their decision, those who *choose* to surrender with dignity. It is a personal decision that is reached by some when they find themselves at this crossroad in life. Only they will understand their reasons.

This group may have a difficult time convincing or explaining to their loved ones how, or why, they reached this decision. For some agreement cannot be easily achieved, surrender is often perceived as *quitting.* Wishes to discuss such things as giving away personal items, or funeral arrangements often cause great upset. Family and friends naturally want the individual to *come to their senses, and accept or continue treatment.* It is important to understand, this is generally a personal decision that is not arrived at lightly, without a lot of soul searching. This pronouncement is generally centered upon an inner voice accompanied by a peaceful sense of surrender, not fear. This group is not to be confused with those who experience a very natural initial panic reaction and sense of doom, which passes. This group is often the very elderly, or individuals with very advanced, and sometimes multiple types of cancer. I will not say always, because sometimes a good pep talk is what is really needed, but in some cases, after careful review, wishes should be respected.

AS DIFFICULT AS IT IS TO BECOME COMFORTABLE WITH THE IDEA OF DEATH, SOMEDAY WE WILL ALL COME FACE TO FACE WITH OUR PHYSICAL MORTALITY; IT IS A NATURAL PART OF LIFE. WHEN WE ARE COMFORTABLE WITH OUR SPIRITUAL IMMORTALITY DEATH IS BUT ANOTHER PART OF LIFE.

Now if we were to conduct a study and the research was based upon 100 participants, all with cancer,(most research study groups are actually much smaller), would we reach the same survival or success rates each time we followed a group for five years? No, because the results would be affected, each and every time, by the number of subjects from each group. Were there more A's than C's? Or more C's than A's. What if they were all A's? What if they were all B and C's? You see how the statistics would change? This is only one example demonstrating if you took a group of people, in this case cancer patients only, there will always be different outcomes. This is because each one of us thinks and acts independently, differently.

These are only three different groups of what may be considered *human factors,* and they are just the tip of the iceberg. Figuring in the human factor, as a variable, is a necessary step in the process of formulating and analyzing any data attempting to predict cancer survival rates. Without a numerical value for this set of variables, the marginal error cannot be established. With no room for error, the results obtained become not much more than fancy guesses.

The missing number lies within the realm of the *human factor,* and here possibilities are stretched almost to infinity and beyond. The human factor is always a dynamic and elusive variable when included in any equation, far beyond just state of mind at a given time. There are countless human factor variables that must be accounted for if we wish to use mathematical equations to produce cancer survivor predictions, and that is without even considering more obvious *physical* matters, such as age, existing health, living conditions and other considerations that may be present at the onset of cancer.

This intangible human factor is a variable that throughout the history of civilization, man has attempted to categorize, and assign numerical values to. To some it is known as human nature. Human nature is so diverse that it would be difficult to even name all of the theories that have been developed through the ages to define us, never mind the number of personal variables that drive each of us. Countless tomes are witness to the devoted efforts of man to define and classify individuals as certain types, to predict behavior. Ideas and observations made by men such as Socrates and Plato, Francis Bacon and Thomas Hobbs, Immanuel Kant, and Georg Wilhelm Friedrich Hegel to Karl Marx, among many others. To this day theories are still being proposed that attempt to establish a way to express human nature and behavior, as a number, through use of categories complete with proper labels. Numbers are essential within equations; numbers are what matters when creating statistics.

IT IS MY HUMBLE OPINION THAT IT IS NOT POSSIBLE TO PRODUCE ACCURATE PREDICTIVE CANCER SURVIVAL STATISTICS THAT ARE BASED UPON OR INVOLVE HUMAN NATURE AND BEHAVIOR AS A VARIABLE.

When it comes to equations involving the human factor as a variable, even if researchers found a way to allow for most of the possible human factor variables discussed, there is yet one even more insurmountable obstacle that will always stymie research analyst in their efforts to assign a numerical value to the human factor; Spirituality, faith, and personal beliefs.

THE STRENGTH OF A HUMAN'S FAITH IN A HIGHER POWER, BE IT FRESH AND STRONG IN THE THROES OF NEW BIRTH OR SURE AND STEADY AS THE AGED OAK TREE, CANNOT BE MEASURED OR ASSIGNED A NUMBER BY MAN.

So why have I carried on at great length with this long winded discussion, regarding something as boring as statistics, when we were in the middle of discussing the fact that you, or a loved one, has recently been diagnosed with cancer? I have carried on to this extent because I want you to remember this discussion as reinforcement against discouragement. We both know that you will no doubt be searching for, finding and reviewing a flood of information regarding your cancer… After all we do live in the age that, as predicted, has *seen learning greatly increased*, especially via internet search engines. I am not saying do not do these searches. For some types and stages of cancer you will find excellent modern, innovative advice and important information about newly developed and discovered advances that can affect treatment decisions. Many of these topics this book will only touch upon the basics of, especially in regards to technology and research. What I am saying is this; Do not let statistical information you may read, regarding your particular cancer at a particular stage, discourage you. Do not accept statistics as full truths carved in stone, as if they are the Gospel, because they are not.

REMEMBER, PREDICTING HUMAN NATURE IS IMPOSSIBLE TO ACCOMPLISH, CANCER SURVIVAL PREDICTIONS, WHICH INVOLVE HUMANNATURE AS A VARIABLE, ARE THEREFORE INHERENTLY FLAWED.

Were you involved in any of the studies that have been produced? Me neither. I read multiple studies that proposed grim survival rates for the cancer I was diagnosed with, at such an advanced stage. As mentioned I was stage IVB. This was especially true due to quality of life concerns because of complications which occurred during and/or after treatment. For example complete inability to swallow was a possibility.

Have you ever heard that saying about the old fool who didn't know it couldn't be done, so he went and did it anyway? Well, that was me, and it could be you too. You have no idea how puzzled, yet how happy my doctors are to see how well I am when I come in for my check ups.

It is also very interesting to note that in early 2011, when I was in for a routine follow up/check up with my radiation doctor, I had to sign a number of documents. I was told this was because of a system wide change in procedure and processing, as well as to gather information for a new study that was under way. Yes, apparently there is a plan underway to release cancer survival statistics that instead of five years will be based upon a two year from diagnosis to *cure*/survival.

Someday we may see headlines generated in Main Stream Media after the scientific world of statistics releases the latest compiled data claiming cancer to have an almost 100% cure rate.   As you journey along the road of *Life During Cancer* do not let other people tell you something can't be done, but don't be led to believe it will be easy either. Be prepared to fight.

IF YOU THINK IT CAN BE DONE, IT CAN. IF YOU THINK IT CAN'T, IT WILL NOT. THAT IS THE KEY, WHAT YOU THINK, WHAT YOU FEEL, WHAT YOU KNOW IN YOUR HEART. IT'S ALL ABOUT A POSITIVE STATE OF MIND.

5 STAGING YOUR CANCER

Staging Your Cancer does contain some annoying yet useful technical terminology used in staging cancer that can be found anywhere, but more importantly this chapter is about trying to make that scary time period between being told you have cancer and jumping right into treatment a little less scary by understanding it a little better.

In the recovery room, awakening from the biopsy took me a little while. The comfortable, foggy floating feeling was so welcoming; I really just wanted to stay in that cocoon like state, safe in the land of no worries as long as I could. You know how it is when the alarm goes off and you *have* to get up, whether to go to work, or school, or just start the day, and it's chilly or pouring outside? How many times have we reached out and slapped that pesky persistent alarm clock into silence via the snooze button a time or two. We know we are going to get up, may even want to get up... but in a minute.

I could hear everything, the conversation, all the little beeps and clicks of machinery in the room, and the whoosh of air pressure released as the nurse at my side finished checking my blood pressure again. I heard her calling me. "Debbie it's time to wake up". I felt her gently but firmly, insistently shaking my arm. I chose to feign deep sleep. I've never thought that ignorance is bliss mind you, but for me, for the moment, it was, and I wanted to hold on to those last few precious moments. Between you and me, I was fully awake. I knew exactly where I was and what was going on, I just wanted those few extra moments of *officially* not knowing if it was real bad. I could blame my lethargy on the fact that I had been exhausted from the past week of worry, and that stress had deprived me of sleep. I could blame it on that, but it would not be the truth. Soon enough I knew I would be getting all of those details that I had been waiting to hear. Soon enough I would know what I was up against. So I allowed myself the luxury of those few additional stolen moments of innocence.

Most of my thoughts revolved around my life before cancer. Random swirling images flitted capriciously behind my closed eye lids. Me when I was strong and active, running, horseback riding, and then on a motorcycle, with the wind streaming in my face, days in the sunshine gardening, rough housing with the grand children. Thinking about how much I loved singing. An ever changing soundtrack of some of my favorite songs played along in a silent chorus that only I could hear, accompanying the images in my head. I knew that when I did decide it was time to wake up that my life, as I had known it thus far, was about to be drastically changed. I took a deep breath and opened my eyes, to face the official staging of my cancer. I would hear all the details.

THERE IS AN ABUNDANT WEALTH OF INFORMATION AVAILABLE REGARDING THE TECHNICAL DETAILS OF CANCER STAGING, THIS IS A REVIEW OF VERY BASIC

INFORMATION, I RECOMMEND THAT YOU DEFER TO THE LITERATURE PRESENTED BY THE EXPERTS IN THE FIELD, AND YOUR DOCTOR.

The following is only a brief overview of accepted standards. It is generally a two step process staging cancers. First is the TNM classification. T stands for tumor, N for lymph node, and M indicates metastasis.

* **T**: Is concerned with the size of your primary tumor and whether or not it has spread to any nearby tissues.
* **N**: Brings into question whether any of your nearby lymph nodes are involved.
* **M**: Determines whether the cancer has spread or *metastasized*, to other regions in your body.

Once these T, N, and M characteristics are known, then stage grouping takes place. This next staging classification system is the one most of us may be more familiar with hearing references to, and it is known as Overall Staging. This is when your cancer will be assigned a final report card which will be based upon a system represented in roman numerals, and generally accompanied by a letter grade of A, B, C, or D.

* **Stage 0**: This is known as carcinoma in situ. This is cancer still in its earliest form. The term in situ means that there is no invasion of radical cells present in any surrounding tissues.
* **Stage I**: This means a Small tumor is present which may be *up to* 2 centimeters in size, and that it is localized in only one part of the body.
* **Stage II:** These are tumors that are *over* 2 centimeters, but generally *no larger* than 5 centimeters. They are considered locally advanced, because of size, but there is still no indication of spread into other tissues or nearby

lymph nodes.

* Stage III: Cancers are also termed as locally advanced, and cancer type can affect whether this stage has been reached. Generally Stage III indicates the cancer has spread beyond the original tumor site, quite commonly to nearby lymph nodes.

* Stage IV: Tumors *larger* than 5 centimeters, and cancer has spread, involving other areas of the body. This may mean that it has crossed tissue barriers, for example moving from fatty tissue into muscle tissue, or bone, or that it is present in distant lymph nodes, or other organs throughout the body.

It is important to note that overall staging and the accompanying letter grades of A, B, C, and D vary greatly and are dependent upon the type of cancer. For example in cases of breast cancer, stage II A the tumor may be *larger* than 2 centimeters and *up to* 5 centimeters, but has still not spread to the axillary lymph nodes. Stage II B the tumor may be *larger* than the 5 centimeter limit, but has still not spread to the axillary lymph nodes.

IT IS ALSO IMPORTANT TO NOTE THAT NOT ALL CANCERS ARE STAGED USING THIS CRITERIA.

For example, forms of leukemia, which affect the blood and bone marrow throughout the body, are not staged based on these factors. Cancers in or around the brain are also not staged using the TNM system, since these cancers tend to spread to other parts of the brain, and not to lymph nodes or other parts of the body.

It is because of the many numerous combinations of possibilities such as these noted, as well as differences of opinions between professionals, that I would defer to the experts. Again I stress, for a more in depth explanation and understanding in regards to the staging of your own personal situation it is recommended speak directly with your doctors, as well as review available literature on the specific cancer type.

What I learned when I did decide to awaken was that I had a tumor composed of malignant Squamous cells, SCC cancer. The tumor itself, about the size of a lumpy malformed golf ball, was a mass that encompassed my larynx or voice box. The good news did not end there though. The main growth had a slim tail that had managed to cross barriers, snaking through layers of muscle and fat tissues approximately two and a half inches long extending downward into my neck. I was classified as stage IV based on size of tumor, over 5 centimeters. Because the cancer had crossed boundaries between tissue types, combined with positive results indicating lymph node involvement, I was bumped into a very advanced stage IVB.

I also learned that any attempt at surgical removal of the tumor would involve complete removal of my voice box because the surgical excision of tumors to remove cancerous tissues generally requires extending the surgery to include healthy tissue. This is necessary to allow a safety *margin*, ensure that all of the cancer has been removed. Since I had such extensive involvement of the surrounding tissues, besides losing my voice box, it was also highly likely I could lose the ability to swallow as well. Due to this I was not considered a good candidate for tumor removal surgery.

With surgery I had a 100% chance that my quality of life would be drastically affected. The voice issue, which realistically state of the art technology offered a very good possibility of regaining speech in the future with a mechanical voice box, was one thing; but the very real threat of losing the ability to swallow was a drastic outlook. Being unable to swallow would be not only life altering, but could be life threatening. Pursuing treatments, as opposed to the surgical procedure, offered the possibility, no matter how slim the percentages were, that I could not only regain my voice, but maintain my ability to swallow. I must confess, my first strong gut reaction was "cut it out". I wanted it gone.

This phase of arguing with the doctors, for me, was almost a mental melt down to be honest. I mean here I was with throat cancer, and I had been privy to similar scenarios twice in my lifetime. I had this overwhelming sense that there was a reason I had been witness to the differences between two treatment courses and their outcomes. You see I have mentioned that my Mom died from this same disease; after the cancer failed to respond to treatment, and had run a long and debilitating course; but there was also Mom's brother, my Uncle Clarence.

Uncle Clarence had throat cancer too, way back in the early seventies. At that time it was pretty much standard procedure to perform surgical removal of the voice box in cases of laryngeal cancers. I remembered Uncle Clarence from when I was a small child. He spoke with a mechanical voice device, and smoked cigarettes through the hole in the front of his throat. Yes, at 8 or so years old that image was pretty graphic, and really stuck with me. My mental dilemma was brought on by the fact that Mom was gone, and Uncle Clarence, even though I have not seen him in quite some time, is now in his 80's, and still with us. I just had so much information to process.

It was the doctor's firm decision to take the no surgical removal route that brought on my temporary melt down. I mean I really thought the message was I needed to do like Uncle Clarence. The doctors were quite firm that treatments were the best route though.

When you are going through this whole diagnosis and staging process before entering treatment, there is just so much information coming at you, and you're scared and unsure of your future it can become hard to think clearly, and make decisions. It's even worse when you make a decision and everyone else tells you you're wrong or that it will not work.

I really did have a lot of doubts regarding whether pursuing treatment instead of surgical excision was the right decision. Based on my faith, my belief in the existence of a Higher Power, I have always felt that things happen for a reason. That being so, I felt that there must be a reason I had been shown in the course of my lifetime two very different outcomes for exactly what I was up against. Mom, who had initially responded to treatment, was gone in two years; yet Uncle Clarence on the other hand, with surgical removal of his cancer, had lived for decades, and even continued to smoke.

I wish I could say that I found the answers I sought in that first mind boggling week of appointment insanity that followed. I wish I could say that I had immediately understood this message to a point I was comfortable with regarding the matter, but I did not. I wavered and worried back and forth between whether the message or the *reason* was focused on the course of treatments chosen, or the outcomes? There were so many questions I had, and so little time to seek the answers before treatment would begin.

I really do believe my Higher Power will never ask more of me than I can bear. For someone who does not believe there is a Higher Power that watches over us, times like these may seem overwhelming. It may be that from a rock bottom point of despair and fear such as facing cancer, that you seek Him. Seek and you shall find.

It is this relationship, whether we are aware of it or not, that is the source of that inner voice that speaks to us, guides us, comforts us and offers strength and wisdom far beyond what we are capable of on our own. I think/feel/accept that my Higher Power is known to many different people by many names, and I Think/feel/accept that we are able to reach out to Him and form personal relationships through different paths.

The Holy Bible can be accurate, and the Living Word, and a source of great comfort, but that does not mean that it is complete. There is a difference. There are no inaccuracies, but there may be omissions. It is wonderful to have the written word of a segment of the existence of man, and his communications with and faith in our Higher Power, but is it not possible that He spoke with others as well? Others who are not included in the Holy Bible? Other "religions" we are not as familiar with? Is there only one right way to "believe"? Could he have created and spoken to others earlier than *the* Adam and Eve most are so familiar with? Why not? For example if your chosen religion is as a Christian, When Cain left Eden he was marked so all would know what he had done, if Adam and Eve were "first", who were the people he was marked to ward off? We argue over His existence, His name, how to properly worship Him, we tell others what to do in His name; we even kill each other in defense of these religious beliefs. All in His name, I find that to be the saddest thing in the whole universe. A relationship with our Higher Power is a personal spiritual one and I would encourage everyone to have an open mind. It is possible to believe all religions and embrace none.

If you do not have your own beliefs, a spiritual relationship, if you do not have faith in something beyond us, I hope you will find it by the end of the journey. If you have no beliefs and are comfortable with that arrangement, then you may perhaps consider my advice as being intuitive and that I am hearing my own sub conscious thoughts. If you are reading purely for information, then read on, the advice is still good; the spiritual faith is totally up to you.

I had faith, I was sure there was a message, but I felt I was missing something. My official staging was accomplished now though, and at stage IV B, the cancer was very advanced, and my doctors wanted treatments begun yesterday. There are many types of cancers that if they are caught at an early stage have very high cure rates. In this case doctors will *want* to move quickly. If the cancer is at a late stage they will *need* to move quickly. Some types of cancer are known to grow slowly, but others may progress swiftly and your doctors will take this into account as well. I had to set aside my questions and doubts regarding what the message could be for the moment, because the present was in my face, here and now, and for the next week straight, demanding my attention.

ONCE YOU HAVE BEEN OFFICIALLY STAGED YOU CAN LIKELY EXPECT THAT THE SHOW IS ABOUT TO GET ON THE ROAD WITH A RAPIDITY THAT WILL MAKE YOUR HEAD SPIN, IF YOU'RE NOT READY AND HOLDING ON TIGHT.

Just after official staging can be a very confusing and frightening time, for the cancer patient, as well as family and friends. Experience has taught me that being prepared for this post staging phase is important. This is the point where you need to begin making your battle plans outlined in the next chapter, *Staging a Plan of Action.*

IF YOU ARE READY YOU CAN NOT ONLY *NOT* BE OVERWHELMED, BUT YOU CAN *ABSORB* MUCH OF THE MASSIVE INPUT OF INFORMATION THAT IS ABOUT TO COME AT YOU WITH AN IMPACT THAT WILL SEEM LIKE THE FORCE AND SPEED OF AN AVALANCHE.

6 STAGING YOUR PLAN OF ACTION

Staging Your Plan of Action is based upon my own personal experience as a stage IVB cancer patient and offers insight into what happens after cancer diagnosis and staging. This chapter takes a look at some of the most common types of cancer treatments, and options as well as a peek into some of my own experiences; such as getting my restraint mask made for radiation treatments, my first impressions of others in advanced stages of treatment, and most importantly this chapter is about how to get organized so that you can be more prepared and ready to do battle than I was, information I wish I already had from day one of diagnosis.

For me the week following staging was very fast paced, passing in a blur with so many things to remember it was impossible. One of the first things decided after diagnosis and staging is usually whether there will be any further surgeries prior to entering treatment. For example will there be an attempt or is there a need to reduce the size of the tumor, or relieve pressure on other structures? In my case while it was decided not to attempt to surgically alter the tumor, the doctors would perform a small surgery to place a PEG tube, this is called a Percutaneous Endoscopic Gastrostomy procedure, and the tube allows liquid nutrition to be pumped directly into the stomach bypassing the throat which in cases of head and neck cancers will undergo changes during radiation treatments that effect swallowing.

After surgical decisions are made focus is upon treatment and the various methods and choices and options best suited to each individual case. Some people may receive radiation treatments or chemotherapy, or may have both as I did.

Radiation treatments have a few different methods of delivery. A close friend's prostate cancer was treated with radioactive seed implants. These are small radioactive surgically and strategically placed seeds that are generally inserted into or very close to the actual cancer site or tumor and they left in the patient. It would probably depend on location but for some prostate cancer cases there is a one day surgery appointment to place the seeds and there are no daily trips as with beam radiation therapy does.

Technology is always advancing and changing, and there are currently external and internal beam radiation treatments in use. My doctors at the time I was treated decided External Beam Therapy would work best in my case.

THERE WILL BE DISCUSSION ABOUT THE CORRECT RADIATION DOSAGE AND HOW MANY TREATMENTS, AND HOW OFTEN, YOU WILL WANT TO NOTE AND REMEMBER.

For Chemotherapy treatments there are many different types of drugs used, of different strengths, and delivery schedules and methods vary widely. Some chemotherapy treatments even come in a pill form. I would be receiving a platinum based agent, which my doctors warned me meant they were "Bringing out the big guns" via intravenous delivery. Some patients will have what is called a port surgically placed for delivery of the chemotherapy agent, which is kind of like a permanent IV outlet. Sometimes the port is placed closer on the body to the cancer location instead of in an arm as one would think. Generally ports are used for patients receiving lengthy or more frequent treatments such as weekly or even daily. This is to avoid the need of putting in a new IV set up at each chemotherapy infusion treatment. It can become difficult in advanced chemotherapy treatment to access veins, as they often become very thin and fragile, and for this reason sometimes these semi permanent ports are used. Chemo drug delivery schedules are administered in cycles and a chemo cycle may be daily, weekly, or monthly. In my case it was decided I would receive my chemotherapy treatment in 3 week cycles.

THERE IS MUCH TO REMEMBER WHEN ALL OF THIS INFORMATION IS COMING AT YOU AND BE SURE TO ASK QUESTIONS AND TAKE NOTES WHILE IT IS.

Any surgeries your doctor determines necessary are generally completed before beginning treatment. This is because cancer treatments such as chemotherapy can inhibit proper healing. The minor surgery for my PEG tube placement was done almost immediately.

Two days later I was back at the cancer center for a second round of input overload. This whirlwind trip included both a tour of the chemotherapy and the radiation facilities in two different but adjoining buildings, and having my radiation treatment mask made. Depending on your cancer type, if you will be receiving radiation treatments, especially of head, neck or throat you will most likely have one of these made as well.

This process was a bit strange and the creation of the radiation mask involved an entire team of very friendly techs who had clearly worked together and done this many times before. They had music playing down low and everyone was like hyping each other up to get it done first try. The atmosphere was like we were at a football game, lots of high fives and smiles. That is me behind it on the cover. I had throat cancer so my motion restraint mask was being made to mold to the exact shape of my head and upper torso including my shoulders and upper rib cage, because during treatments besides the actual tumor some distant lymph nodes were being lined up for targeting as well. The radiation treatment mask is created using a very rigid mesh like plastic material that has locking plastic set ups along the outer edges. This hard piece of plastic is heated up to a certain point and for a very short time becomes soft and pliable, able to be smoothly molded over the body part it is placed upon, such as a head. The mesh composition allows for breathing with the mask in place. The last thing you will see before you close your eyes is the team gently and evenly dropping a warm net like rubbery cloth down upon your face. Mine was light yellow colored. Once that warm soft mesh settles into place all hands are on deck as the tech team works quickly gently but firmly pushing and molding every nook and cranny, eyelids, nose, chin, and jaw line into perfect conformity; if they take too long and the plastic hardens then they must start all over again with a fresh piece.

The plastic material was quite warm when it came down and covered my face, but in no way hot enough to burn or cause any pain. I wasn't constrained at that point so it was kind of like getting a warm facial massage to be honest. I had really long hair in pony tail, and it had been pulled off to the side so that my head could lay flat on the table. Even though my eyes were closed, it was a comical moment when the whole team at about the halfway done point got to the mass of hair and almost panicked, quickly conferring with each other as the clock ticked and the plastic hardened, "what to do with the pony tail?" They decided to swoop it up towards the top and slightly off to one side and they molded a hole for the tail to exit. Because of the resulting hairstyle they cracked jokes that I would be the Krissy "Winter Precipitation" of Winship (copyright friction?)... For those old enough to know who that was and the hairstyle connection, it was funny, until I lost my hair later on in treatment.

The radiation mask when completed and cooled into rigidity would be placed over my face and chest and attached to the treatment table by the corresponding lock set ups and enforce complete and absolute immobility. This was the most difficult part of radiation treatments to get used to, those few moments each day being locked into place. Completely immobilized and tightly restrained. I understood the mask was to ensure my head and upper torso remained perfectly still in place on the treatment table so that the tumor and lymph nodes were lined up with the track of the computer programmed radiation beams, but it did not make it any easier.

The machine used for my external beam radiation treatments was quite similar to an MRI, but a lot bigger. If unfamiliar it is sort of a tube shape or tunnel that the table the patient lays on slides into. It is very important to remain perfectly still while the dosage is being delivered, even to the point of trying not to swallow. This is why small children are often sedated for radiation treatments.

At my very first "lock down" radiation treatment simulation trial, as they were working their way around clicking the five locking clips into place with the little tool they used to do it, Click! Click! Click! It was taking a little while, the locks are tight when the mask is fresh, Click! Click! I admit it, I couldn't help it, I panicked and had to be released. It was so absolutely immobilizing. The team was very quick to comply and it was reassuring how fast they got me out. The techs let me get my composure and psyche myself back up before we tried again. I did manage to get the hang of relaxing and accepting the confinement, kind of, but it was not easy.

At this point I had just barely completed my first week post diagnosis and stress levels were already on the way up. I had been through biopsy and PEG Tube Placement surgeries, had my treatment mask made, and had been through introductions to the three doctors who would make up my oncology team, a radiology oncologist, a chemotherapy oncologist and an ENT (Ear Nose Throat Specialist). There was also a blurring procession of staff, the doctor's nurses who you can come to with questions and the interns in training, crisis coordinators and councilors from the facility and support group representatives for patients and for caregivers. Each doctor discussed at great length the treatment that they would be responsible for and we were given opportunities to ask questions at every meeting. I remember my husband and I were just so shell shocked, trying to take it all in, not even sure yet how we were going to manage this everyday daily routine. Every time we were asked "do you have any questions"? We just kept saying "I guess we just have to trust you and follow the schedule". It was the end of October and we met with the receptionists after all the meetings and I was set up with appointments that stretched into January of the following year.

I stressed about the fact that I felt like I was already growing weary from the daily running to appointments. I was only one week into this and was already becoming unsure of my ability to keep this pace up for much longer. The first time I walked into the radiation treatment waiting area had had a strong impact on me. The walls were lined with rows of matching well padded taupe colored chairs, complimented by two of the softest, cushiest sofas in the world. These were grouped around a very impressive focal point, an immense aquarium/terrarium set up that was open for viewing from both sides. When we had arrived promptly at 10:00 a.m. that day, every available spot was filled with people. The waiting area was packed. Seeing the patients in there that day, when I joined them for my first treatment had suddenly made cancer feel much more real, scarier, like nothing else had up to that point. Some were the family and friends who brought them, but most of the seats were filled with people like me, people with cancer. These people were not like me though, I had walked in there. Many of these people were very sick with cancer at different stages and points in treatment. Most had little or no hair at all. I was especially struck by the children, many with brain cancers and often heavily sedated or very weak. I was shocked seeing the physical condition of some of these patients. Many of them were in very advanced states of debilitation, emaciated, lethargic, slumped in chairs or parked along the wall on a stretcher. I had not really felt much fear up to that point, but walking into that waiting room absolutely terrified me. I could look like them in one month, or two.

We were out the door early each morning, while it was still freezing outside to make the 75 mile drive to

Atlanta, and then after the daily appointments back in the car and drive all the way back home again. Often we would leave before light and arrive home after dark. I knew I would be doing this every day, except Saturday and Sunday, for many weeks. Even though the radiation treatments had not been too bad, up till this point, changes within my throat and mouth were already becoming apparent. If only one week of treatments had these effects, how bad would things be after 6 weeks passed? Not to mention I had not even begun chemotherapy treatments yet.

    I worried a lot about that first upcoming chemo cycle I would be doing the next day. The radiation treatments had been trying, and took some getting used to, if you could call it that. They were so far bearable after managing to convince myself that I could pretend I was a yoga master. I could go to my happy place, my quiet little lake, well more like a pond, and make myself lay perfectly still under the stiff restraint for the ten minutes or so at a time. I became pretty good at pretending I was watching the breeze chase the clouds, or the play of sunlight on the water. I was really afraid of the chemotherapy for some reason though. Terrified would probably be a more accurate description. After only one week I was already on the verge of freaking out and having doubts.

    I was trying to figure out what to wear for the big chemo day, and rummaging in my closet for the hoodie I wanted, thinking about just how long the day I was facing would be. The chemo cycle would take eight hours they said, as long as a full day at work. I was supposed to go for my radiation treatment first, down to the bat cave as we had nick named the cavernous nether reaches of the radiology radiation treatment unit located in the Winship Cancer Center's Tunnel level. Afterwards I was then to go to the main level chemo lounge as it was called. Part of those 8 hours I would be receiving hydration and anti nausea medications through the intravenous drip, but at some point the steady drop of clear fluids would change. Then the little drip, drip, drips, would become the toxic, platinum based chemotherapy agent, which would enter my veins, drop by drop. I was wishing I had a laptop, wondering what should I bring, a book, snacks, drinks, would I need the cell phone charger? I was getting pretty frustrated trying to find the hoodie that I wanted. It was November, just really getting into the cold spell here in the south, and I dug deeper into the closet.

That was when my hand closed upon a strangely familiar feeling item. It was an old well worn and scarred black leather back pack. Long ago in my youth it had accompanied me across thousands of miles and through countless adventures in my younger days as an avid biker. This was an item that had been stored for almost a couple decades now; my chaps and old scuffed up Bell half helmet were laying next to it. With my hand still gripping the pliant well used and abused leather bag, the inner voice said quite clearly *you need this*.

That was the moment when what I can only describe as an epiphany or vision of sorts hit me. It struck in a mental flood littered with bits and pieces of intertwined images and thoughts from the past and present and even me in the future. With the force of a tsunami wave it washed over me, and when it had passed, all doubts and fears I had been feeling were washed away, and I felt infused with sense of strength and confidence that remained and carried me through the next months ahead and into the future. I had a plan of action.

While on my knees, with my face buried deep in the warming folds, engulfed by the pungent aroma of seasoned leather a silent movie of seemingly unrelated images played out at very high speed. Perhaps another time, another story, I will someday attempt to better explain the details of this very intense experience. What was important was what I took away from it. I remember it began simply as I realized what I had grabbed and was just kind of sentimentally swept away, remembering good health and good times on bike trips, wind in my hair, but then I was seeing people and scenery flashing by. Some of the people were wasted away and others I saw rushed into emergency rooms, I saw one at home in bed turning off an alarm clock, I saw so many people passing in a blur crying, laughing, arguing, hugging and loving, living and dying. What I learned from those moments on my knees in the closet with that old leather black back pack is very hard to explain, but the important part of it as I understood it that relates to entering cancer treatment so that others can know, *before* going through a hectic exhausting first week of life with cancer like the one I had just been through is what is most important. If you let them the treatments can kill you as quick as the cancer.

IT'S NOT JUST ABOUT SURVIVING THE CANCER; IT'S ALSO ABOUT SURVIVING THE TREATMENT AND A BIG PART OF WINNING THE BATTLE AGAINST CANCER IS ORGANIZATION WHICH WILL REDUCE STRESS.

Cancer treatments are going to be your new job, your new school, your new daily routine, it can be an exhausting ordeal and absence is not allowed. You will not be paid in dollar amounts for going to work each day, you will not get a better grade on your report card, what you can expect are positive results reached by setting a goal, and sticking with it. Chapter six will go into a much greater depth regarding tips to achieving these goals, as well as why this mind set approach to treatments is of such great importance. What matters for now is that you understand from the very start, it will be hard, you will need a support system, you will need to be organized and you will need all the help and encouragement you can get to survive the treatment plan.

APPROACH YOUR BATTLE AGAINST CANCER NOT WITH FEAR, BUT WITH PREPAREDNESS, ORGANIZATION AND CONFIDENCE.

Sounds great you say, so how do I do that? To begin with, get yourself a back pack. No ladies, large pocket books will not do. It must be a backpack. You want a big roomy one, with at least a couple of inner or outer zipper pouches for storage separation, which will allow easy access for things like cell phones, keys, glasses, pens, parking stubs, medicines, etc... Don't worry that your backpack may not be quite as symbolic for you as mine was to me, or if it looks empty at the start of your journey, give it time, it will fill, and your attachment to it will grow.

Picking out a back pack, or getting one for a friend is a big step towards preparing. To be prepared we must be organized. Believe it or not this back pack and its contents will in many ways become your base of operations over the next few months, mine did. Be sure your backpack choice is sturdy, with comfortably well padded shoulder straps, and zipper pockets.

AT THE START OF THE JOURNEY STOCK YOUR BACKPACK WITH THESE SIMPLE THINGS:

A 3 SUBJECT NOTEBOOK, AN ADDRESS NOTEBOOK (PREFERABLY BOTH OF THESE WITH FOLDER POCKETS), A CALENDAR, A FEW PENS, AND TWO DIFFERENT COLOR HIGHLIGHTER MARKERS.

The three subject notebook is to provide a section for communications between you and each of your doctors. Whether it is questions you want to remember to ask, or answers, instructions or advice your doctor has given that you want to remember, there is a place for them. The smaller notebook will be for your own personal notes you may wish to make, and for writing down contact information for friends you will make along the way. The calendar will become your organization focal point, your Companion Calendar.

In the early stages of diagnosis, and as you are whisked through staging, and meeting doctors, and barraged with input regarding treatment plans as I was, this little tip will help you maintain your sanity. With so much to remember it's great to have an organized place to put everything. It took me a week of playing catch up since I didn't start out with my back pack. The backpack will serve early on as a receptacle for all of the informative brochures, schedules, the blood work results that you will be requesting, instruction sheets, sometimes samples from your doctor's offices, water bottles, surgical masks, laptops, books, you will be amazed at all of the things that will go in the back pack along the way; and how glad you are to have it.

At the moment you are probably a bit skeptical, and you are thinking seriously, a simple back pack is going to help save me? I tell you yes, not all by itself of course, but, it will help. Believe me by the time you finish your very last treatment, after you have gone for a few follow up visits with good reports; it will be really hard to break the habit of having it with you. When I finally decided to stop bringing my black back pack, and re-retired it, I felt like I was putting away a comforting teddy bear I had outgrown.

Now that you are aware of the importance of the Back Pack and that you should it have right after diagnosis and staging, and filled it with its simple contents, let's jump right into organizing your companion calendar.

Here we will share tips and tricks that hopefully help make life with cancer just a little more bearable for everyone.

7 GOING THE DISTANCE IN THE TREATMENT COURSE

Diagnosis may have been arranged through referrals from your primary care physician; therefore treatments are not necessarily undertaken at the same hospital as diagnosis takes place. *Going the Distance* is a broad look at approaching the overall treatment period, including options such as where you may choose to undergo cancer treatment, from home base or at a cancer treatment facility that offers in house. There are also support resources. This chapter encompasses the idea that, for a time, life will be revolving around a very strict schedule that must be followed. It is about wrapping your mind around the enormity of this fact as a whole. About making the abnormalities in life that must be endured, seem just a little more normal. Chapter 8 *Keeping a Light on at the end of the Tunnel*, will discuss day to day coping tips and tricks to help ease the journey, including everyday issues of emotional and physical natures; from pain and frustration, to nausea and constipation, as well as maintaining nutrition, hydration and a sense of humor, but *Going the Distance* is about understanding what's coming, how best to handle it, and establishing new habits, and a new routine.

THE MAJORITY OF US, NO MATTER WHAT AGE WE ARE, WILL OPERATE BEST AND BE MOST COMFORTABLE WITH SOMEWHAT OF A ROUTINE.

We all have our own little quirks and habits, responsibilities and goals that together comprise our day to day living routine. Our own personal orbit that has a gravitational field we know and follow. Cancer is like a meteor unexpectedly sideswiping us, bumping us just enough to alter our course, and settle us into a new orbit.

Entering treatment for cancer temporarily shatters all of our normal and comfortable daily rituals and activities with a stomach dropping jolt. I felt like I had just completed this colossal, intricate jigsaw puzzle that took me years to complete, and while I was still in the process of straightening up, stepping back to admire the completed masterpiece, enjoying the last few satisfying cracks from the vertebra in my back, and exhaling a sigh of satisfaction, some stranger came along in the breath of a nano-second, and swept it off of the table, onto the floor. We must accept that this has happened, and set about picking up the pieces and putting the puzzle back together.

Aside from providing the recommended web support resources, before proceeding with the creation of the companion calendar, I feel mention of *away* from home treatment options should be included at this point. The recommended websites provided will also be very useful in researching these options. It is even possible to communicate with other cancer patients and find firsthand accounts and opinions about specific facilities that you may be interested in. You will still want to complete your companion calendar even if the *away from home* option is preferred because many cancer care centers that do provide living facilities will require a companion present. Also most patients who stay will plan weekend trips home.

Where to go for treatment is a major decision every cancer patient faces. I chose to go to a cancer center because quite frankly it is so much easier when all of your appointments and doctors operate within one facility, smoothly, as a team. All inclusive cancer centers such as the one I went to are becoming more and more popular, and can be found associated with and operating within many of the larger city and state run hospitals, as well as completely independently. You will need to make inquiries in your area. Due to copyright law in this edition I refrain from recommendation to any particular facility, and limit mentioning by name only to where I myself sought treatment. Having such a well equipped one stop facility available is wonderful, but sometimes, as in the case of my Mom, who lived in tiny little Burke, New York, facilities such as this are not always a choice or an option, and the in house option is a fairly recent development within the past few years.

Some patients must go to one place for radiation, another for chemo, as well as maintain a primary care physician to oversee general health. This was the first choice I was given, if I wanted to keep treatments in nearby Newnan. In this case it will take greater organizational skills, strong patient participation, and perhaps a little extra patience. Trust and establishing excellent communication between the doctors, making them truly work as a team, is a must. With organization this can be a can do.

IF YOU HAVE NO CANCER CENTER CLOSE ENOUGH TO TRAVEL TO, AND YOU FEEL ARRANGING DOCTORS AT DIFFERENT FACILITIES WOULD BE TOO DIFFICULT, YOU MAY WANT TO LOOK INTO CANCER CARE CENTER OFFERRING AN INPATIENT OPTION.

For example I did briefly consider going to a cancer treatment center in another state. I would have been closer to my two daughters, and my best friend. I chose to stick with my original wish to stay *home* for treatments, and decided upon Winship in Atlanta. Even at Winship we qualified by meeting the over 60 mile distance requirement, and were offered the choice of using the apartment facilities, called Hope House. This *home away from home* was available for their cancer patients. Like many other Cancer Centers these arrangements included, and even encourage/require a caregiver/companion to accompany the patient. This is why a companion calendar is still a great idea, but travel and stress will be greatly reduced with this arrangement. Most offer communal kitchen/living room apartments with separate sleeping quarters, as well as convenient shuttle services to provide transportation between treatments and Housing Facilities.

For some people, especially those who enjoy traveling, this *away from home* treatment plan could actually be a quite attractive arrangement. The other reason someone may want to consider an away from home stay at a cancer center's facilities is as I mentioned, there may be a facility in a city or state that is closer to more family. Again, personal decision, and of course costs and insurance issues will play a role in deciding.

I chose to pursue treatment from the home base because I have never been a big traveler; I am quite the home body. All of my animals were at home, my parrot, my boxers, my horses and my cats and yes even my chickens and rabbits. I liked the comforting normalcy, the feeling there was still a natural order that I associated with simple things. I like waking up to the sound of a rooster's crowing as he greets and welcomes each new day. Everything *normal* for me was at home, and I wanted to stay home. I wanted as much normal as I could get. My husband was the one who had insisted on viewing Hope House, and wanted to keep it open as an option. He was the one who kept renewing our place on the waiting list. You will need to inquire regarding specialized Cancer Care facilities in your area but;

THE OPTION TO CHANGE TO IN PATIENT STATUS WILL GENERALLY BE AVAILABLE AS LONG AS A PATIENT'S NAME IS RENEWED WEEKLY ON THE LIST; IF TRAVEL BECOMES DIFFICULT, DUE TO HEALTH OR WINTER CONDITIONS, THIS IS A VERY GOOD OPTION TO HAVE.

I say this back up is a good option to have because as noted, cancer type, location, stage, as well as current physical condition will all be deciding factors not only used to determine the treatment plan that will work best for each individual, but how each individual holds up through those treatments chosen. At a few of my low points I had to be carried to the car, and used a wheelchair to maneuver through the buildings. At my lowest I spent seven days admitted to the hospital weighing less than 90 pounds. We may see that one person only needs to receive radiation treatments, another may receive only chemotherapy, while yet others, like I did, will get the double whammy, and do both. All of these important indicators will play a major role in just how bumpy the ride will get while going the distance in the treatment course. Trust me we had days when my husband said "That's it, I'm checking you in at Hope House so you're closer to the hospital."

THE LEVEL OF DIFFICULTIES ENCOUNTERED AND THE CHANCES OF COMPLICATIONS DURING TREATMENT RISE OR FALL DEPENDENT ON A COMBINATION FACTORS SUCH AS CANCER TYPE, STAGE, LOCATION, TREATMENTS, AND OVERALL HEALTH.

Working with the information that has been presented thus far, now is the time to aggressively, not passively, but aggressively organize. Get your ducks in row. Whether it is you yourself with cancer, your child, your parent, your better half, or your best friend, setting up a personal companion calendar, one that meshes with the treatment schedule will prove beneficial.

TWO OF THE BIGGEST SETBACKS ENCOUNTERED BY THOSE UNDERGOING A RIGOROUS CANCER TREATMENT REGIME ARE STRESS AND MISSED APPOINTMENTS; THE GOAL IS TO REDUCE BOTH THROUGH ORGANIZATION.

As a cancer patient individuals may feel everything is coming at them too fast. Treatments can affect energy levels, and cause a sensation of being overwhelmed, that things are moving beyond control. To caregivers what may seem like simple discussion about who's driving tomorrow or the next day or next week, can sound more like a debate to the patient. This can be especially so when conversation turns to topics that include conflicting schedules, such as childcare or work, or a forgotten special event that is going to be missed. Sometimes these discussions can create or reinforce a sense of being *indebted* and *dependent,* a *burden.* This can be detrimental to the cancer warrior. What's up the next day, or *the next* discussions, can cause enough frustration to make the patient upset, throw their hands up, give in and give up control or participation.

AS A WARRIOR YOU WANT TO FEEL ABLE TO MAINTAIN REASONABLE CONTROL, TO CONTINUE TO PARTICIPATE; AS THE CAREGIVER PART OF YOUR DIVERSIFIED SUPPORT ROLE IS TO HELP THEM ACCOMPLISH THIS.

In the course of the ensuing whirlwind that most are whisked through after diagnosis you have been given many details. At the end of your first week if you were ready your backpack will no doubt have a number of brochures, instruction sheets, prescriptions, etc. I know mine was pretty plump. Hopefully your three subject notebook, which you divided by categories to suit your needs, has been helpful. I divided mine by doctors; my ENT surgeon, my medical chemotherapy oncologist and my radiation oncologist you can suit yours to your needs. This notebook hopefully now contains responses to many questions that have been answered by your doctors, as well as advice they have offered, and an expected treatment schedule. These notes will be useful in setting up your calendar.

YOUR TREATMENT SCHEDULE WILL BE BASED UPON YOUR NEEDS, AND WHAT YOU HAVE TO DO NOW IS SCHEDULE YOUR LIFE AROUND MEETING THESE NEEDS.

For some life may be quite lonely, and filling a calendar may seem impossible because you may think there are not many who will be able to help. There are still a number of places to turn that can offer resources, encouragement and support if this is the case. These places can not only help fill in empty squares left in the calendar, but can help fill voids in your emotional needs and your heart as well.

IN THE LIFE OR DEATH STRUGGLE, IN THE BATTLE AGAINST CANCER, EVEN THE LONELIEST OF PEOPLE WILL SUDDENLY FIND OUT THEY ARE NOT ALONE.

Whether you go to church, or you have never thought about it at all, whether you attend or belong to a particular local church, almost all will be very welcoming. Here you can find compassion, and most have a wide variety of community outreach and volunteer organization programs that can offer help. There are also a number of social service organizations available that can provide important services such as transportation and companion / caregivers on a volunteer basis.

It is very important to have back up and encouragement; this is true whether you are the person with cancer, or the person who loves someone with cancer. This is why I have included the next two vital resources.

Whether you are having difficulty filling all of the treatment days on your companion calendar or not, a good support group can be a blessing when trying to locate additional needed cancer care resources. Whether you are the cancer patient, whether you have plenty of friends and family in your life or not, whether you are the family member or friend that is in the companion/caregiver role.

SUPPORT GROUPS OFFER AN EXCELLENT SOURCE OF INFORMATION AND ENCOURAGEMENT, AS WELL AS ASSISTANCE LOCATING VITAL RESOURCES.

You will find that many hospitals and cancer centers offer a variety of cancer support groups. Generally these meet on a weekly or monthly schedule. These groups can be great if as a cancer patient you feel well enough to be mobile during treatment, and as a caregiver you can find the time. Besides travel problems though, there is another problem connecting with kindred spirits at these local, smaller support groups. Since there are so many types of cancers, so many stages and different treatment plans, it can be difficult to meet someone that you really relate to within the smaller groups. Someone in the same boat so to speak. For those who are computer savvy though there is a whole world out there, and it is a much easier matter to reach out and connect.

Through reputable, well established websites fellow cancer patients and their caregivers can interact and share at a worldwide and on a local level. There is a virtual treasure trove of information, support and encouragement available that is literally at your finger tips. I highly recommend the following two websites that I have used personally, and still frequent to this day; they are a must have resource for the cancer patient, as well as family and friend caregivers.

BOTH WEB ADDRESSES SHOULD BE INCLUDED IN YOUR ADDRESS BOOK AS A VALUABLE RESOURCE.

My first favorite, as far as information in one place is The American Cancer Society. This website is accessible at WWW.cancer.org, and if you think you need help filling your calendar as far as travel and companionship you will definitely want to go here. The American Cancer Society not only has forums for caregivers and cancer patients to form friendships and receive advice, but also provides many convenient direct links. These links are easy access to valuable information and resources. From non-profits, government, state and local level resources and programs, to clinical trials information that may be available as well. Through use of search option directives results can be narrowed, for example to a specific geographic location or cancer type. There is also an extensive, reputable collection of cancer literature from experts and researchers available here as well.

The second site I would like to recommend is my personal favorite. At Inspire you will find real people dealing with real cancer issues. I preferred Inspire as my main resource for forming friendship and finding advice, not only from the level of been there done that, but support and encouragement from people that were doing it right now, right along with me. The web address for this resource is world wide web inspire.com, and a search for Paaatriot101 will still find me and I do still log on every so often to inspire and offer encouragement to others in treatment.

Now that you have this additional information, as far as where to look for companion/travel assistance if needed, and choices regarding where to go for treatment, it is now time to fill in the treatment period on the companion calendar. This window of treatment period whether tackled from home, or away, begins from the start of treatments, through completion, and ideally should include an additional period of a minimum of at least one month. This additional, somewhat more flexible window, allows for assistance and companionship through the first few weeks after treatment ends, which as discussed further in chapter 9 *Cut Loose* can be a very difficult time.

For each treatment the doctors will discuss how long they can be anticipated to last, as well as what can *generally* be expected during the course of each treatment plan. Do not be afraid to ask questions throughout that stage. That is what your bigger notebook is for, questions and answers between you and your doctor that you will need to review when setting up your companion calendar. The medical chemotherapy oncologist will also provide literature outlining specific effects related to or associated with certain types of chemo agents, as well as a calendar explaining the cycle schedule chosen.

Armed with a predicted *window of treatment*, you will signify these days in your address/calendar book with your lightest colored highlighter marker. I used yellow and red; so first my calendar showed my entire treatment course highlighted in yellow.

The next step is to review all of the notes from doctors that need to be taken into consideration when setting up your *companion calendar*. As discussed schedules and strengths of the chemo agents that could be used vary greatly. This is an important factor that should be discussed with your doctor, and notes taken.

THERE ARE USUALLY EXPECTED "BAD" DAYS IN THE COURSE OF MANY CHEMOTHERAPY CYCLES, DEPENDENT UPON AGENT USED, FOLLOWED BY "GOOD" DAYS. BE SURE TO QUESTION YOUR DOCTOR ABOUT THIS.

How do you know when you can expect good days? Ask your doctor. If you are on a 3 week chemo cycle for example as I was, your doctor may say, day one through three, take your nausea medications as ordered, and expect that you are going to be sick as a dog; he may also say that you can expect to feel better over the course of a two week period. This would mean that one week out of the three *less help* might be needed, but for at least one week to two weeks out of the three, *more help* will be needed.

On your calendar that has the entire duration marked out, you will want to add this information. The "bad" days you will want to highlight with the second marker. For example I used yellow for the duration, and red to highlight anticipated bad days. Red + yellow = orange Meaning full time assistance most likely required. The color scheme does not matter, for example yellow + blue = Green could mean full time assistance. The important thing is that travel appointments, such as chemo delivery days and expected accompanying "bad" days, extra help days, are able to be easily identified.

Radiation treatments, unlike many of the chemo agents, are almost always *every day*. Sometimes, especially in cases involving children, who must receive smaller doses, these treatments are broken up into more than one treatment per day. If the doctor has ordered radiation treatments, the schedule, realistically, from mask fitting and simulation to completing treatments, could span up to two months of every day except Saturday and Sunday, just like going to work. Monday through Friday you will be going to appointments. Each of these appointments will probably average less than half an hour of time when things are running smoothly. You must allow for travel to and fro though, and understand sometimes there will be delays, as well as Dr's appointments which are usually at least once per week per doctor. Depending on drive time, radiation treatments can amount to a very substantial and taxing chunk out of the day.

In my case I began experiencing severe headaches, nauseousness and almost narcoleptic fatigue within an hour of coming out of treatments by the time I began my fourth week of radiation treatments. So, even though I had bounced back somewhat from my first round of chemotherapy, there was no way I could have even considered at all even in an emergency safely attempting to drive myself at all by the end of the first month.

Depending on individual circumstances there may not be a need to use the second highlighter color, indicating full time assistance at all, or not until completing a portion of treatments. The organization and planning of the companion calendar is geared towards acknowledging there will be ups and downs in the treatment course, and expecting them, and accommodating them.

One of the biggest differences between radiation treatments and chemotherapy is how and when they affect the cancer patient. Chemo nauseousness may set in almost immediately; it may subside and resume, passing from bad days to good days. The effects of radiation treatments are much more subtle as they settle in. These may include symptoms such as the possibility of areas of skin burning, serious oral health and swallowing concerns, especially in cases of head and neck cancers, as well as pain from damage and/or swelling and edema of surrounding tissues within the field of treatment. While the radiation treatment itself does not hurt, there can be damage to surrounding tissue and bone as a result of the almost microwave like processes involved with external beam therapy. These types of symptoms may be expected to generally worsen as treatment progresses.

I HAVE READ IN MULTIPLE SOURCES THAT AFFECTED TUMOR AREAS TARGETED WITHIN THE LINE OF EXTERNAL BEAM RADIATION TREATMENTS CAN CONTINUE TO "COOK" FOR MONTHS AFTER TREATMENTS HAVE ENDED.

As noted earlier some cancers, such as leukemia's and specifically blood cancers for example, are not treated with radiation, in that case chemo would be the treatment of choice.

WHILE BOTH RADIATION AND CHEMOTHERAPY TREATMENTS ARE WIDELY ACCEPTED AS CONVENTIONAL METHODS IN CONTEMPORARY SOCIETY TODAY FOR MANY FORMS OF CANCER, THESE TREATMENTS ARE TOXIC BY NATURE.

It is because of this that in most cases it is likely there will be cumulative effects upon the body, of one kind or another, over time. These may include compromised immunity, lowered energy levels, and impaired abilities, as well as development of symptoms that require pain management.

IN OTHER WORDS, TO PUT IT SIMPLY, THE INDIVIDUAL BATTLING CANCER, ESPECIALLY AT ADVANCED STAGES, WILL NEED HELP.

For some people, and some cancers, the treatments may not be quite so intimidating. For example in the course of my treatment regime, just shortly after completing my second cycle of the platinum based agent, I met an elderly lady, 69 years young who was doing once monthly chemo cycles. This woman was there for her third round of treatments, and had just returned from vacation. She said she felt great, and she certainly looked wonderful. I must confess, as sick as I was at that point, after my second round with *the big guns*, I was quite jealous. A friend treated for prostate cancer seemed to sail right through his treatment. In his case the doctors used radioactive seed implants. Another dear friend, despite all efforts ranging from surgery to chemo and radiation therapy succumbed to pancreatic cancer. I was stage IVB only a couple of letters from the worst it can get, and I am still here. As I have said and cannot stress enough there are many types of cancers, different strengths of chemotherapy agents and radiation therapy delivery methods, each case is as going to be as individual as we are.

WHAT MATTERS IS THAT WE UNDERSTAND THAT WHILE THE EFFECTS OF TREATMENTS VARY GREATLY, PRIOR KNOWLEDGE AND ORGANIZATION CAN HELP EASE THE BAD DAYS, AND HOPEFULLY INCREASE THE GOOD DAYS.

Once it is determined when, how much and how long help will be needed, it's time to start working on filling in your help wanted companion/caregiver vacancies.

THERE SHOULD BE A RECOVERY PERIOD OF A MINIMUM FOUR WEEKS AFTER TREATMENTS END INCLUDED IN THESE PLANS AS WELL.

Section III will discuss the post treatment period in greater detail, but it is important to remember when setting up the companion/caregiver calendar be sure to include arrangements for assistance extending into this crucial period. It may also be helpful to note that under the guidelines of the Family and Medical Leave Act (FMLA) it is possible for family members to be granted leave time. This program allows for much greater flexibility in cancer treatment situations involving for example a spouse or child. The program is operated by the; U.S. Department of Labor Wage and Hour Division (WHD). You should inquire regarding available benefits and confirm details directly through the human resources department at your place of employment.

That being said, let the calls begin. You can choose to do this yourself, or as a group tag team effort. You may have someone you trust who is especially talented at organizing details that you would like to appoint. It is up to you. Call all of your friends and family members, and let them know what you're up against. Of course your close, current friends and immediate family will no doubt be chipping in, but don't stop the calls there. Many are honored to be asked, and actually appreciate knowing in advance specific dates help will be needed.

FILLING IN THE COMPANION CALENDAR WILL GUARANTEE YOU HAVE THE COMPANIONSHIP, SUPPORT AND TRANSPORTATION YOU NEED WITH THE LEAST AMOUNT OF STRESS... AND IT COULD BE FUN CALLING OLD FRIENDS.

For me my help was my husband, my four grown children, one close friend, and friends of friends, but there are many ways to fill the gaps in the hedge, and some can be fun. Call Aunts and Uncles cousins and nephews that you usually only see at Thanksgiving or Christmas. You can call old high school friends that you haven't seen in years, college dorm buddies, or current fellow students or co workers.

When making the calls, after explaining the situation and how many weeks treatment will last, extend the invitation to come and share a few days or a week of the adventure. Let them know the dates and ask if there is a period that would be best for them. Let them know the real deal in advance. You may not be the best of company; quite frankly you may very well go through periods that you are, to be blunt, bitchy. You need people around you who understand this and will not become easily offended and choose to leave. There may be down times when you need positive people around you to encourage and assist, emotionally, spiritually and physically. Be honest when you call, tell them you would like them to share a part of this important journey you are about to undertake. This organization and advance planning can make a big difference.

For example in my case my daughter Tennille was with me four weeks, but we scheduled the weeks scattered over a period of three months. Some weeks my husband would work, and local friends would arrive early in the morning, bring me for appointments, and stay until Kevin came home at night. My other children came a week each too. Between family and friends we actually ended up with more people ready to come and stay for a week than we had weeks, and a couple weeks our empty nests was chirping with activity as visitors overlapped. As I went through the progression of the treatments, which became ever so much more trying and tiring as they went on, seeing old friends, my children and my grandchildren was such a blessing, and they really did keep me going and motivated. When life deals you lemons, make lemonade.

THE TREATMENT PERIOD CAN BE RIGOROUS AND FRAUGHT WITH PERILS AND PITFALLS, BUT IT CAN ALSO BE A TIME TO STRENGTHEN OR RENEW OLD BONDS, AS WELL AS FORM NEW ONES.

While you are making calls if you have chores that need doing work out delegating these to volunteers during this process as well. For example in my case I had chickens and horses that had to be fed and watered twice a day and brought in and out because it was the winter months while I was in treatment. This work was included and divided on a weekly basis between my son, two neighbors and my husband. Everyone knew when they were expected to fill in.

As you go through your list you should also assign a few flexible *back up* people that can warm the bench, and be ready to pinch hit if there is a glitch in the plans, a hitch to the giddy up. When I had finished we had filled 12 weeks of my calendar with a rotating cast of characters. These were the people who would stick by me, put up with me, and look out for me throughout the next few months.

Names and contact numbers of each confirmed companion went into the address book, and friends and family filled the days on my calendar. Instead of looking at the calendar, counting days to the end of radiation treatments or checking how close the next dreaded chemo session was, I looked at the calendar and thought; "Oh awesome I'll be seeing my grandsons next week", or "Ooh three more days till Kris comes with my granddaughters", or "Meg is coming and she is so lively and brightens anyone's day" or even "What fun next month will be catching up with my best friend Laura, who lives over a thousand miles away".

I do recall in the course of treatments there were a few surprise changes in scheduled companions. These took place   smoothly and in stride. Make a list with everyone's phone numbers and dates expected and give one to everyone in your circle. There was no stress over details like so and so has a cold, and should not accompany me to treatments over the next few days as planned. Oh no what do we do? It was covered, there was open communication between caregivers. Not everyone who is going through cancer treatments will need so much help. Some may need more, some may need less. This chapter has been about preparation, getting ready to embark on a journey in the; the next chapter is devoted to doing it.

Keeping *The Light at the End of the Tunnel in Sight* will focus upon predictable and often preventable mental and physical challenges that may be encountered while in treatment. Here Observations and advice, from the bird's eye view perspective of the cancer patient, as well as the caregiver, come together.

Whether you are the cancer patient/Cancer Warrior, or a tribe member/companion/caregiver, you can gain a better understanding of what to expect; the good, the bad, and the ugly. You can gain knowledge and information, learned in hindsight by others who have been there done that, geared towards recognition and prevention of important factors that can affect health, happiness or quality of life. Topics such as nutrition and dehydration, concerns such as sadness or anger, frustration and depression, are discussed in depth; from the patient standpoint, as well as the caregiver's.

INFORMATION ABOUT PREVENTING THE PREVENTABLE AND COPING WITH THE UNAVOIDABLE COULD HELP SAVE A LIFE OR A RELATIONSHIP.

8 KEEPING THE LIGHT AT THE END OF THE TUNNEL IN SIGHT

This chapter is about coping with and when possible avoiding some of the more common pitfalls; Fatigue, stress, dehydration, malnutrition, depression and yes even anger and arguments that may arise in the course of that critical phase of *"Life During Cancer"*, the time while actively receiving cancer treatment. Here the tips and advice touch upon aspects and/or perspectives of cancer treatment perhaps overlooked or lesser known in medical circles. Topics range from; recognizing the real importance and value of achieving proper rest, nutrition and hydration, maintaining regular bowel movement evacuations and even regaining out of control emotions. This chapter is about *keeping that light on at the end of the tunnel* while getting through the treatments. Why the tunnel comparison for this chapter? Many who receive radiation treatments will find that these facilities are often located below ground level, hence tunnel. The Light represents hope which springs eternal.

When I Look back now upon my own cancer treatment period, which involved external beam radiation treatments every day, combined with a platinum based chemotherapy agent administered in three week cycles, with appointments scattered between for three different doctors, week after week after week, at first glance it really seems like it wasn't that bad at all. Funny how time can do that to painful memories isn't it? Women can probably relate better to that, it is like going through childbirth, the pain was excruciating, it was real, but over time the memory fades.

The prolonged eviction process to dislodge and remove the squamous cell cancer that had taken up residency in my throat was a hard fought battle, brutally won at a cost that is still being paid to this day. I know there were horrible earaches and severe headaches, as well as excruciating pain endured preceding, accompanying, and following each and every swallow for a time. But I kept on swallowing. I remember the seemingly endless days of vomiting that for me struck within hours of completing the first round of chemotherapy. I know there were days I was weak and helpless as a newborn kitten. I went through bouts of dehydration and suffered poor nutrition absorption. I shed most of the muscle mass that I used to be so proud of, dropping well below the 100 lb weakling mark during treatment. Pain and doubts were among my constant companions, but luckily not my only company as I worked my way through treatments; weeks passed into months marked day by day on my companion calendar with organized time spent with friends and family as scheduled in advance.

Remember get that *Companion Calendar* set up, it could be one of the most important things totally within your power that helps improve your survival chances simply by reducing stress.

STRESS, EVEN WHEN AN INDIVIDUAL IS HEALTHY AND IN PRIME PHYSICAL CONDITION, CAN BE DEBILITATING.

My intention with the brief dire description of my own treatment period was not to scare anyone, remember as noted earlier individual circumstances will vary greatly depending on many factors; cancer type, stage, age and treatment choices and options, I was merely trying to explain what treatment could be like to help prepare you. Hope for the best but prepare for the worst you know. For example during my treatment since swallowing ability was affected I supplemented what I was able to eat orally with a liquid nutrition that was pumped through the PEG (Percutaneous endoscopic gastrostomy) tube directly into my stomach. Not all cancers involve the throat or impact swallowing though so therefore some situations may not require that measure.

There were some days that were not so bad, but there were also those other days that I felt totally and absolutely helpless. On some of *those* days, even though at first I protested being treated like a baby, I ended up carried to the car and tucked in for the drive to Atlanta. On those days I had to use a wheel chair and get pushed around in the hospital to treatments and appointments. I became one of those people from the waiting room that had scared me so badly. Many individuals like me are not real good at first asking for help; sometimes we can even be quite stubborn about admitting weakness or the need help or accepting it graciously when it is offered.

CAREGIVERS KNOW WHEN TO IGNORE THE WAVE OF THE HAND AND THE INFAMOUS "I GOT IT" WHEN OFFERING ASSISTANCE.

I can tell you there were at least a couple of occasions that my caregivers kept my stubborn I can do it all by myself self from falling down.

CANCER WARRIORS SHOULD BE GRACIOUS AND ACCEPT AN OFFERED STEADYING HAND, ESPECIALLY ON STAIRS.

Sometimes even if we think "we got it", blood pressure spikes or drops, medications, not eating well, etc… any of these could bring on an unexpected wave of nauseousness or dizziness and better safe than sorry is a good motto.

CAREGIVERS SHOULD BE ALERT FOR SIGNS OF FATIGUE OR WEAKNESS INDICATING HELPING HAND NEEDS TO EXTEND TO HANDS ON; ALWAYS BE PREPARED TO SUPPORT FULL BODY WEIGHT TO PREVENT FALLS.

There came a point about 2 months into my treatment that I was in such rough shape, down to 86 pounds, I was admitted through emergency as an inpatient to the hospital by my radiation oncologist. I was put in an isolation ward, and could not even receive flowers. This was because I was suffering leucopenia; a dangerous lowering of white blood cells which meant my body's defenses that were supposed to guard against germs and diseases was down. This can be a dangerous side effect during chemo and/or radiation therapy treatments and is one of the reasons you can expect your doctors will order blood work tests often through-out the course of treatment. Keep that in mind when you reach that point midway through treatment when you feel like a pin cushion… just remember it is for a good reason. I also remember at one point I had to supplement potassium because testing revealed it was dangerously low. Potassium is important for kidney function. Remember also to ask for a copy of your test results as you move through treatment.

YOU CAN EXPECT THAT BLOODWORK WILL BE DONE VERY OFTEN THROUGHOUT TREATMENT, THIS IS NORMAL.

I didn't want to be admitted, I hated being confined anywhere for any amount of time. Most of me was just so tired and weak at that point for the first few days after they rushed me in I really did not even care or think about that I was there at all. After a few days rest, when I was more alert, I actually appreciated the break from the grueling daily routine we had established for a little bit, but I really considered the time spent inpatient as a more of a break for my companion caregivers than myself though. During my week as a patient I was brought to the tunnel every day for my radiation treatments on a stretcher. After a week though I was ready to get home again and let everyone know it.

Luckily I went through this episode without contracting a cold or flu bug or worse developing the dreaded pneumonia. I had actually been using surgical masks through most of my treatments, because I had been warned my immunities would be very low during the chemo cycles, and being winter I worried about catching colds when I was in public, especially closed in elevators. At first in stores when I was still getting around people would look at me funny, but then I made stickers to put on my masks, they said "I am not contagious, I Just have cancer". That seemed to help cut down on people yanking small children away from me.

DURING CHEMOTHERAPY TREATMENTS WHEN OUT IN PUBLIC PLACES, ESPECIALLY DURING COLD AND FLU SEASON, WEARING A MASK AND WASHING HANDS OFTEN IS A GOOD IDEA TO HELP PROTECT FROM INFECTIONS WHILE IMMUNITY LEVELS ARE LOW.

As I mentioned because we had to travel we had to be awake by 5 A.M., dressed and out into the cold winter weather by 6:00 A.M. to battle traffic on the almost 2 hour trip to Atlanta. Some days there were only the radiation treatments to get through, which from check in time to done and out the door on the occasional smooth day could be as quick as one hour, but on a glitch day, when the schedule is running behind due to equipment failures or patient situations this could stretch 2-3 hours before we could make the drive back home. We had some days we were home as early as 2:00 in the afternoon if there were no additional tests or blood work or appointments scheduled, other days if I had tests or appointments with doctors scheduled, which happened often, we did not make it back home and in the door until well after dark. Chemo cycle days it was usually after 8:00 P.M. at night before we were home.

It is the day after day after day of this demanding schedule that can get to you and wear you down. Getting enough rest and sleep is very important because your body rejuvenates while it is at rest sleeping. I am not saying stay in bed, exercise and fresh air and having interest in the goings on around you are always good, I am just saying keep in mind you want to be sure to allow enough real sleeping and resting time. I was bad at first about catching forty winks when I had the opportunity, it seemed weird to be taking a nap in the middle of the day. I got over that after the first couple weeks of treatment though. I learned that a little moderation and prevention can go a long way preserving energy levels. It just wasn't worth wearing myself out trying to do overly strenuous or stimulating activities, and those little rest periods here and there prove beneficial in the long run.

NOT ALL CANCERS HAVE SUCH A RIGOROUS TREATMENT COURSE; TAKE EXTRA PRECAUTIONS THOUGH TO KEEP STRENGTH UP AND STAY STRONG.

You may think well I've been diagnosed with cancer obviously I'm not going anywhere…. well you would be surprised how many people make all kinds of plans when they find out they have cancer. The unspoken, in case I don't make it attitude… Or I have cancer I'm going to do what I want to do. I knew people that did things like traveling to California to see Hollywood in real life, another friend decided to make the rounds across country visiting family and friends, incorporating side trips to major casinos along the way. I am not saying do nothing I am just saying personally I would strongly recommend that from the point treatment begins to avoid over doing it and keep your focus on treatment.

DON'T WAIT UNTIL EXHAUSTED TO REST, GET INTO THE HABIT OF RESTING WHEN ABLE; THE CELLS IN OUR BODY REJUVINATE DURING SLEEP. THIS ADVICE GOES FOR CANCER WARRIORS AND THEIR COMPANION CAREGIVERS.

For those undergoing radiation treatments you must also take care of your skin within the target zone. Radiation treatments can cause a reaction that creates burns on your skin ranging from mild sunburn to extremely severe blistering burns. The more severe burning when not related specifically to a very rare equipment/mechanical issue is generally because of lack of routine moisturizing. Ask your doctor about this early on so that if possible you can begin a moisturizing regiment before you even begin treatments like I did. My doctors prescribed a cream but I had a very large Aloe Vera plant that I cut leaves from to express the gel like contents and used that. There is a very good reason so many hydrating lotions and shampoos claim the benefits of aloe vera, because it works. I began using the aloe gel about a week prior to actually beginning treatments and continued throughout and for some time beyond completing them. I do realize everyone cannot find an aloe vera plant, and I am sure your medical professionals will provide a cream to use, but I wanted to mention this because the doctors were quite impressed at just how well the natural remedy seemed to work at keeping the burning to a minimum.

SPEAK WITH YOUR RADIOLOGY ONCOLOGIST ABOUT SKIN CREAM FOR MOISTURIZING RADIATION TREATMENT AREA AND USE REGULARLY AS DIRECTED.

Proper Nutrition, ugh I can still remember shuddering at the mere thought or mention of food. I used to hate coming in through the A wing of the Hospital when I had to see my ENT (Ear, Nose Throat) oncology guy because the cafeteria was right there and I had to go past the food aromas, coffee and frying eggs and sausages and toasting breads in the mornings, and at lunch time even worse… The food smells would even follow me into the elevators. Some days it was all I could do just to hold it down and keep it together, with my face smothered down into the chest of my hoodie or buried in the leathery aroma of my backpack. Within private space such as at home or in a car there is a lot more control over smells and odors, but when out and about it can be a challenge. Many everyday smells encountered may seem cloying, heavy, nauseating or feel overpowering. This can happen in restaurants or near crowds where people are wearing heavy perfumes, even when exposed to some cleaning agent odors. During treatment we can become very sensitive to scents. Often these exposures brief or prolonged can ruin an already very fragile appetite because stomach acids get to churning in response to certain trigger aromas.

ADD TO YOUR BACKPACK A SCARF / KERCHIEF/BANDANNA AND A LIGHT NATURAL SCENT (POWDER/SPRAY) KNOWN TO BE BEARABLE/PREFERABLE FOR USE COUNTERACTING OFFENSIVE ODORS WHEN OVERWHELMED.

Aside from general nauseousness and trigger aromas negatively impacting appetite during cancer treatments there are additional issues as well, such as changes with how the taste buds themselves perceive foods, which can be quite extreme. The condition even has a fancy name, Dysgeusia. If you have a head/neck/throat cancer and will be receiving radiation treatments within that target area you can pretty much expect to experience taste changes, as well as a decrease in salivary production, and a difference in textures, or the way foods feel in your mouth to occur. Many chemotherapy agents used to treat a variety of cancers can also affect tastes and salivary gland function, from the mild to the extreme.

WHETHER RECEIVING CHEMOTHERAPY, RADIATION THERAPY, OR BOTH CHANGES WITHIN THE ORAL CAVITY WHICH IMPACT EATING WILL LIKELY BE ENCOUNTERED.

I have always been a pretty simple basic eater; eat to live not live to eat. I never ate a lot of to go or restaurant food, I favored vegetables and fruits and my biggest goody sin was and remains ice cream, so, when the doctors and nurses told me I could probably expect changes in flavors and a "metallic aftertaste" when eating or drinking certain foods, especially sugars and sweets I thought "no big deal" right? Boy was I wrong; it was a real big deal. I am a pretty tough old bird, and in my entire life there have been very few occasions that I have ever broken down and cried, I rarely shed a tear over anything trivial, but I admit it, I bawled my eyes out twice during treatment, and both times were over food. I am actually smiling as I recall it here for you, but at the time I remember clearly I was like totally devastated (smiling broader now).

The first time was the very next morning after my initial chemotherapy treatment. I was exhausted, my face was so swollen I looked like someone else. I had thrown up all night and all the different medications I was on had me feeling so tired and yucky and here we were up and getting ready as usual, early, cold A.M. for the trip to Atlanta for radiation treatments, and I was handed my first morning cup of coffee. As ill as I was I reached for it with such great anticipation. It was my lifesaver, it was going to get me moving, it was my normalcy in a world gone crazy, my precious fresh ground beans, beloved coffee…. and I took a big deep greedy first sip…… and promptly sent a spraying misting mocha Java Joe geyser airborne. It tasted disgusting! Clumsily getting up as fast as I could, waving my arms wildly "look out coming through" I stumbled/ran for the kitchen sink, gagging and heaving and bawling through it all "I can't even enjoy my coffee" waaaaaaaaaaa! Yes I had a serious melt down over my coffee that day.

I really never did figure out what metallic taste the medical profession people were talking about… I did not taste metal, and quite frankly no one else I have spoken with describes the effects on tastes like that either. It is very difficult to explain because while true many taste buds do seem to lose sensitivity, for example the sweet sensors, the remaining sensors seem extra sensitive to other tastes like bitterness. All I know is you never knew what something was going to really taste like until it was in your mouth. Telling me my taste buds and reactions would revert to that of a very small infant experiencing new tastes as baby food is introduced in a high chair, and that I would even be spitting food back out would have been a lot more accurate than "you might experience a metallic taste". Some things were more bearable simply because I was able to at least recognize the base taste of them, while others just tasted plain horrible yuck. There had been minor changes up to that point from the radiation treatments, I couldn't taste sweets as much and I had almost no saliva, but until that chemotherapy treatment I had still been doing pretty good eating various things like mashed potatoes and gravy, and my coffee though more bitter, had been bearable. After adjusting my coffee to no sugar at all and brewing it stronger I was at least able to drink, if not enjoy, my coffee after that day. During treatment you too will find your go to and stay away foods. Will all chemo agents be like that? Many patients report taste changes and/or loss of appetite, but I think it was the type of chemo I had, the "Big Guns" platinum based stuff. I can tell you for sure my sense of taste was severely impacted, but I did not taste metal. It was very frustrating you just never knew if you were going to be like "mmm good", able to stand it or "yuck disgusting". I recall I tried some pineapple chunks at one point, I thought they were going to be good in the natural juices, I was wrong and ended up spitting them out too. Sugars, sweets, yuck, but I was pleasantly surprised to recognize the taste of asparagus and squash varieties with a bit of pepper and hint of butter.

AVOIDING SUGARY FOODS IS GOOD BECAUSE CANCER CELLS LIKE SUGARS AND TEETHARE MORE PRONE TO DECAY DUE TO DRY MOUTH DURING/AFTER TREATMENTS.

So it is actually a good thing foods with high sugar content tend to taste the worst and become the most unrecognizable. Simple but nutritionally fulfilling foods such as Oatmeal or eggs scrambled with a little salt and pepper were not bad. Also I found many vegetables, especially green ones, which are better for you anyway, remained recognizable. We ate a lot of salads while I was in treatment, and still do.

EXPECT TASTE CHANGES, EXPERIMENT WITH FOODS, DO NOT STOP EATING, YOU MAY BE SURPRISED AT SOME OF THE ODD THINGS YOU FIND YOU ENJOY.

There are also a number of nutritional supplement drinks available, which can be pumped through a PEG Tube like the one I had, or drank normally. Some of them, in some circumstances will be covered by insurance. I had problems keeping down two of these brands, and copyright rules will not permit me to say the names of the nutritional drinks, but perhaps in a later edition if there is a response to the enquiry made to the company is received I will be able to include this information; frankly they should be backing my book and "Boosting" my sales because our insurance company didn't want to cover the cost, although they would pay for the other two. We fought and won because even my doctors noted that I had problems with the other two. I did a lot better holding down the one, and if you really need to drink a nutritional drink, of the choices available, it does taste better… more importantly the texture was palatable. It is hard to explain politely, but let me just say the other nutritional supplement drinks felt kind of slimy to me and leave it at that.

I personally found maintaining nutrition with the taste and textures issues to be experimented with and overcome much more of a challenge and quite frankly more important to overall health than how much water I drank, but most people during the course of cancer treatments will find that those within the medical profession involved in their care tend to push the importance of hydration. That is because hydration is very important for a number of bodily functions even in the most normal of conditions, so needless to say if we are going to be flooding said body with toxins and chemicals on a daily basis it is a really good idea to keep up water intake.

INTAKE OF ADEQUATE FLUIDS AND MAINTAINING PROPER HYDRATION HELPS THE BODY FLUSH TOXINS.

Unfortunately all too often when nauseousness is present water seems to be the first thing many are willing to pass on. Cancer treatments are not the same as babying yourself through the night in the case of a brief stomach bug, a short lived flu or a bad meal. You cannot get by with a little ginger ale and crackers, cancer treatments often cover extended periods of time. This is why it is so important to continue to stay aware of and maintain hydration levels to the best of your ability throughout. I know because I remember being "bugged" by my companion caregivers about drinking more water. I don't just mean they bugged me to drink, I mean I was bugged about them bugging me. Kind of became a sore point with me to be honest, even though I had the PEG tube and could use it for water as well if I wanted to, I felt the water seemed to increase nauseousness. I mean really sometimes I just wanted to curl up and be left in my misery. They would be checking my water bottle levels to make sure I was drinking enough, and I would be dumping off some here and there just so they would leave me alone, thinking I drank more than I did. Got to where they tried to sneak in and shoot some water into my belly while I was napping through the PEG tube. We did learn one thing from them trying to get away with that… the cold water woke me right up and definitely did increase nauseousness. After my clothes and bed sheets were changed and all the vomit was cleaned up I realized why I awakened and immediately threw up (they did feel bad). We learned very slightly warming the water and/or nutritional supplement to body temperature reduced the nauseousness. After they learned about that little trick they did get better at occasionally sneaking in some extra H2o. I ended up with a Feeding Pump, a pumping station that had to go everywhere with me for hours at a time. It was electric/battery operated and on a wheeled pole, with a bag that is loaded with the nutritional supplement drink. The contents are then released slowly in very small timed drips and the stomach is so slowly fed it does not notice (Theoretically). Basically it was like an IV set up, but it delivered to my stomach.

TRY KEEPING DRINKING WATER AT ROOM TEMPERTAURE OR CLOSE TO BODY TEMPERATURE TO HELP REDUCE AND/OR PREVENT CHILLED WATER NAUSEA.

I thought the medical personnel were kind of redundant on the topic of drink water, in hindsight though I had to agree with them. Even though I really thought I had managed to keep up a fairly good daily intake of water, during the point when I was admitted to the hospital under emergency circumstances for that one week they said I was seriously dehydrated. Both of my arms frustrated the efforts of many experts to get an intravenous line started in a vein. Everyone had about given up, we had sprayed blood round about more than once, and they had all begun seriously eyeing the larger veins in my neck when Doctor B my favorite doctor who was my radiation oncologist (and also happens to be active military Reserves Hoooahh) came in and he got it done. That was the talk of the hospital all week, and all the nurses loved him because no one could recall the last time they ever saw a doctor jump in and do something as low level as start an IV line, not to mention how efficient and professional he was after they had all but given up.

SEVERE DEHYDRATION MAKES IT MORE DIFFICULT TO LOCATE AND "HIT" VEINS FORLAB TEST BLOOD DRAWS AND/OR IN THE CASE OF EMERGENCY TO DELIVER MEDICATIONS.

Maintaining good oral health and preventing tooth decay is another challenge faced by many during cancer treatments and yet another reason drinking water often is important. The cells in our mouth regenerate the quickest, and because cancer treatments kill cells, with no distinction between good and bad, oral cavity health is often impacted during cancer treatments. The limited saliva that is produced tends to be very thick and can feel almost like ropy strands that are hard to clear from your throat. During treatment and for some time beyond a condition known as mucositosis or mucositis may be present. This can be a result of chemotherapy and/or radiation treatments and result in the formation of very painful sores and blisters to form. Mucositosis can become so bad it can even affect the gastrointestinal tract. I cannot stress enough how important oral care really is, during treatment and far beyond. Rinses of salt water and Baking soda are usually recommended throughout to help maintain cleanliness and PH Balance. Pain in the mouth and throat due to development of sores can be quite intense, especially by the time treatments end. A prescription used by many of us was called magic mouth wash by most of the doctors. It was a slightly numbing and antibacterial solution with a very thick consistency. I found it way too thick and yuck tasting as was out of the bottle to gargle with, but I did use it during treatment and for almost a full year beyond treatment after using water to dilute it to a slightly thinner consistency.

ASK YOUR DOCTOR ABOUT THE PRESCRIPTION KNOWN AS MAGIC MOUTHWASH ANTI BACTERIAL NUMBING RINSE IF NOT OFFERED.

To be healthy the mouth or oral cavity needs to be moist, but during cancer treatments when salivary production is reduced dry mouth can become very extreme. Sometimes this can be so bad that it results in discomfort. For example mouth sores may form because of dry lips and/or inner cheeks sticking to dry teeth. Gingivitis and/or gum problems can develop, and over time a dry mouth environment could contribute to tooth decay. Another problem is that the saliva produced is very thick, and can feel almost like stringy strands in your throat. It can be difficult to clear the mouth and throat of the thickened saliva, leaving one with an uncomfortable almost choking sensation and always having a sense of something in your throat that needs clearing, so you cough more. This offers little relief though, because the thick sticky strands just move up and down slightly, but remain stuck to the sides of the throat. This sounds gross, but I am going to highlight, it is worth keeping in mind because this thick saliva can be a long term problem.

COUGH THE IRRITATING SALIVARY ROPES UP ONTO THE BACK OF YOUR TONGUE, STICK TONGUE OUT, USING DRY NAPKIN SCOOP AND REMOVE.

Often you will literally almost feel like you are pulling long strands of hair up out of your throat. It is such a relieving feeling when the throat is cleared.

There are products on the market made for dry mouth, and even if I did want to mention brand names to be honest there were and are none that I would highly recommend. I found most of these products to be too heavy in both taste and texture when all I wanted was moisture. I had a bit of an edge as a country girl with an herb garden at my disposal though, and I did partake often of my green teas because they seemed to be beneficial to me in many ways especially maintaining oral health. I made a mix of Stevia, persimmon leaf, mint and honeysuckle. I feel green teas are good for you and I already knew that the Stevia plant, which has a number of benefits, was also believed to be beneficial to oral health; Stevia has been an ingredient in mouthwashes and toothpastes in other countries, like the EU and Japan for many years.

ORAL HEALTH CAN BE ENDANGERED BY DRY MOUTH ENVIRONMENT KEEP DRINKING WATER ON HAND AT ALL TIMES AND BRUSH TEETH OFTEN.

Lastly staying hydrated is also important as an aid to maintaining regular bowel movements as well. Trust me the importance of pooping regularly is probably the least openly discussed and the most highly underrated. While in the course of cancer treatments many patients will be prescribed pain medications which by themselves are often associated with encouraging constipation, but diet changes and decreased physical activity levels can affect regularity as well. Right from the start of cancer treatments my doctors were highly recommending that I begin using laxative supplement on a daily basis. I wanted to avoid resorting to using these over the counter remedies long term because I felt that daily use could lead to more problems down the road, such as becoming too dependent on them.

IRREGULARITY, MISSING BOWEL MOVEMENTS CAN CAUSE A NUMBER OF PROBLEMS FROM GRUMPINESS TO PAINFUL STOMACH ACHES AND/OR VOMITING AND IN SEVERE CASES HOSPITALIZATION.

When on pain management medications the normal warning bells indicating that a stomach ache may be a much more serious symptom of impending impaction could be overlooked, ignored or even mistakenly treated with additional pain medication, which masks the pain. Sometimes inadvertently too many days can pass without really even being aware or noticing that so many bowel movements have been missed, until it becomes serious. When confronted with serious stomach pain you should be able to answer the question "When was your last bowel movement" within a reasonable timeframe.

MAKE NOTE OF THE REGULARITY OF AND/OR MISSED BOWEL MOVEMENTS.

Most doctors agree there is no set standard for what is or is not regular, but many consider less than three bowel movements per week to be borderline constipation. There are stories of people going ten days or more without pooping, and for them it is normal, and there are others who say they must go every day, or even multiple times. Some go in the morning, some go at night. We all have our own normal and the goal should be to stick to your normal. If you've had an existing problem with irregularity, then hopefully one of the tips that follow will help you find your "regular".

Either way, at your preferred time, get into the habit of at least making the effort. For me it was always and remains in the morning along with my coffee. All through treatments I would wake up an hour earlier than I needed to, just so I could have my quiet time without being rushed. More importantly though I learned to use that private time on the throne as an opportunity to enjoy a few quiet Zen moments and engage in light beneficial exercises. In cancer treatment or not, anyone can try some of the following tips geared towards relaxation, light exercise and which may encourage bowel movement regularity.

The combined length of the small and large intestines in the average adult are over 20 feet long, and these lie within the belly in looping coils. What we eat is ingested into our stomach and then our body extracts the nutritional elements as it moves along the intestinal tract, and along the way it transitions from one four letter word to another; going in as food and eventually coming out as poop. We do not want it to move too fast (diarrhea) because then our body would not leech out sufficient amounts of good nutritional matter, and we do not want it to move too slowly or we could get backed up and have belly aches and hold in toxic waste build up.

In the intestines there are rhythmic contractions, which we don't really feel that constantly keep things in motion, moving waste forward along the way. Take into consideration the words rhythmic contractions. Emotional upheavals and upset stomachs, constipation and/or straining over stools, pain medications, slumped constricting posture, or curling up into a ball or fetal position in misery, etc… can all serve to disrupt this rhythm. You want to give all those feet of intestines all wrapped up inside the opportunity to relax and do their job. If they get out of rhythm try a few totally relaxed, quiet, Zen moments and see if it helps get things back into sync. Ever heard that old saying about feeling like your stomach is tied up in knots? Could be this is what they meant.

CREATE OPPORTUNITIES FOR UNINTERRUPTED QUIET TIME ALONE TO RELAX NOT ONLY THE ABDOMINAL AREA BUT THE MIND AND BODY AS WELL.

There are a number of very simple relaxation techniques that I stumbled across as I blindly found my way through the "regularity" aspects of life during cancer treatments. Some of these tips are just plain common sense and others discovered accidently through trial and error because they felt good, for example belly puffing. Posture tends to suffer when we don't feel well and often tired cancer warriors will find themselves in a somewhat slumped position for extended periods of time if sitting, or curled up into a fetal position in bed. This can cause compression in the abdominal area and restrict natural actions of the intestines. We all know how to suck our bellies in when we want to look thinner? Well try puffing your belly out instead. I found that quite often I would actually feel movement of fecal matter and/or gas as soon as the constriction was lifted by giving my intestines a little more breathing room.

PUFF/SWELL BELLY OUTWARDS, COUNT TO TEN, RELEASE, REPEAT.

An important thing to remember is that these quiet private moments, besides possibly helping to encourage regular bowel movement activity through relaxation, can also be beneficial to other body parts as well, such as lungs, mind and muscles.

During cancer treatments it can be very difficult to remain as physically active as we would like to or as we should be. When engaged in an exceptionally difficult battle against cancer, in the midst of the pain and bone tired fatigue the very idea of having any energy at all to do exercises seems preposterous and out of the question. I would have laughed at someone, or maybe told them to get lost, if they came to me beyond my fourth week of treatments talking about "hey I have some exercises I want you to try". It is even funnier when you consider that while these exercises can be done anytime and anywhere during the day used as a relaxation technique, I am encouraging you to do these exercises in the bathroom while sitting on your porcelain throne. Some of these might seem a little silly, but don't knock it till you try it, you may be surprised.

First I would recommend controlled deep breathing exercises, which are geared not only towards relaxation and achieving a bowel movement but also to encourage lung health. Your lungs are very important, and when we are sick or not feeling well, when confined to flat out bed rest, there is a tendency, without even realizing it, to breathe much more shallowly than we normally would. This is not good for the lungs, especially over a prolonged period of time. During cancer treatments many are not as likely to engage in heavy or prolonged activity that would increase adrenaline flow, which would in turn elicit a response to inhale deeply, expanding the lungs to capacity as additional oxygen is pulled in to meet the bodily demands of the physical exertion. In cancer treatment while we may not be able to drop and give twenty push-ups or run a mile in two minutes, we can exercise our lungs by remembering to expand them, to stretch them out to capacity once in a while.

EXERCISE YOUR LUNGS: INHALE SLOWLY, UPON REACHING MAXIMUM INTAKE STOP BRIEFLY, AND THEN PULL IN A BIT MORE AIR, HOLD 3-5 SECONDS, RELEASE SLOWLY, EXHALING THROUGH TIGHTLY PURSED LIPS COMPLETELY.

I would also recommend reaching/stretching exercises. This one is very easy to do, sitting or standing, and trust me it may sound silly, but it feels good afterwards. Feel free to use visual techniques to encourage really reaching. Maybe your special place is in an orchard with a tempting bright shiny red apple under a canopy of sun gilded green leaves just beyond your grasp? Perhaps your visual is a basketball court and you're reaching for the hoop to make that slam dunk? It could even be outside beneath the stars far above, reaching and stretching for the brightest one you see.

TRY TO REMEMBER AT LEAST ONCE A DAY TO DO A FEW STRETCH REPETITIONS. ALTERNATE LEFT AND RIGHT ARMS, REACHING, REACHING, REACHING… AND HOLD FOR THREE SECONDS, REPEAT.

Massaging various pressure points on your feet I found can also be quite pleasant and bring about some surprising results. There is probably an abundance of literature available regarding Ancient Chinese medicine and pressure points and how they can affect bodily functions, but this tip is another of those I kind of stumbled across, although I had "heard" a little bit about pressure points before. Many people may have heard or read somewhere that firmly applying pressure on the webbing between your thumb and index finger could relieve headaches? I did not have as much luck with relief using that one as I did massaging my feet. Besides, who doesn't like a good foot massage?

WHILE MASSAGING FIRMLY AROUND THE BACK AND FRONT OF ANKLES "I" OFTEN EXPERIENCED A RELAXING EFFECT ON MY STOMACH.

I have of course no scientific support of a connection between feet and digestion, but it seemed to work for me, so it is worth giving a try. I think many old health remedies may be highly under rated to be honest.

There is no scientific support for this either, but I did also listen to tones I produced using crystal glass, similar to the sounds of Tibetan healing bowls. This was because I had read from multiple sources that claimed the sound or tone of 528 Hz helped repair DNA. Again there is no scientific evidence supporting this, but I want to share what I did accurately. I used an old antique crystal goblet I already had that I felt was producing the correct sound when compared with samples from videos online. Have you ever heard of anyone filling glasses with different levels of water and producing music? I did it like that. I believe only true crystal puts out the ringing tones. This is something you may research further, again I am only mentioning because I want to share what I did, and as long as it does no harm…. I do still to this day occasionally rub my crystal and produce the tone.

I think relaxation moments are important. Nicely inform your companions/caregivers that you would like total privacy for a little while when you are seeking your Zen moment, maybe even get a little do not disturb sign. It is either that or do like I finally did and get mad. I realized how much I needed my private time, but nicely saying "Please do not bother me when I am in the bathroom" wasn't working… I finally resorted to yelling my response "leave me alone for at least a half an hour from now on when I'm trying to poop!" They got the hint after a couple times. I mean seriously I sound mean, but I really wasn't. I did nicely try to explain how much I wanted that alone time. I know they meant well, but I would be just finding my Zen moment and "knock, knock, knock", on the door… "Are you okay?"

You may have seen a comedy show or two that have done skits about getting grumpy when constipated? I know I have. This is kind of a funny truism. Real truth be told though, Cancer Warriors can get grumpy, we can get emotional, and we can develop what may seem like odd or eccentric behaviors over the course of making it through the cancer treatment period; whether we stay regular or not. Outbursts, conflict of interests and yes believe it or not outright arguments, even among the closest of friends and family members can and do happen sometimes no matter how hard we try not to.

For example when riding with my husband driving those first few weeks he would often ask if he could stop and grab a breakfast sandwich and I would say yes, but only because I felt bad if he had to go hungry. I would be crabby the rest of the ride though, and for hours afterward, because the smells upset my already always unhappy stomach. I started getting irritated that he even asked about food and in my mind I no longer cared if he went hungry; I mean really? I can't enjoy eating so why should you? Couldn't you think of eating something at home before we got in the car? Like a smell free bowl of cereal or something? I felt like the first time or two was no big deal… but he already knew food smells made me feel sick, so in my mind if he really cared he would not keep asking. I finally got mad and by about the fourth time the blow up happened. Instead of just nicely rolling my eyes and sighing "oh go ahead" when he asked if could he stop I started yelling at him and ended up letting out all the anger I had been holding in. What part of I find the smells of food nauseating did you miss? Do you not understand it is especially overwhelming locked up in a car with it? Like it was his fault I couldn't eat and I didn't mean to be but I was jealous seeing others "enjoying" food in front of me. Of course the poor man, exhausted himself, had some choice comebacks. We both ended up yelling and I ended up in tears. By the ride home we both apologized, he was sorry and said he should have realized and I was sorry and said I should have just told him I couldn't stand it and it wasn't his fault I didn't like food anymore.

DO NOT WAIT UNTIL BLOW UPS HAPPEN OVER MINOR ISSUES, IF SOMETHING BOTHERS YOU SPEAK UP. SAY "I AM VERY SORRY I KNOW I AM A PAIN IN THE BUTT, BUT I REALLY CANNOT STAND THIS OR THAT"

It is a little easier to understand emotional outbursts and get past them when we take into account what caused them; Stress, fear, exhaustion, uncertainty, changes in habits and health, etc… Everyone has their own way of handling hard times, some of us when the going gets rough literally get tough, others take it in stride and always have a smile ready and some will withdraw and need more encouragement than others. Moods can change rapidly and or drastically depending on each of us as individuals, or sometimes what day of the week it is or what time of day it is, or how something tasted or if we pooped or not. We can get touchy, emotional and grumpy at times, here's a little secret you can use sparingly as needed:

EMOTIONAL OUTBURST CAN HAPPEN;WHEN ALL ELSE FAILS BLAME IT ON THE *STUPID CANCER*, PLAY THAT *I'VE GOT CANCER CARD*, DO NOT PASS GO, GO STRAIGHT TO FORGIVENESS AND HUGS ALL AROUND.

Treatment time can be very stressful for everyone involved, the patient and the companion/caregivers who love them. Being over tired is in general not good for anyone, but being tired, concerned over the success or failure of the treatment course embarked upon, life or death, making it to all of those treatments and doctors appointments, combined with the daily responsibilities and routines of keeping household and finances up and running is very stressful even for the individual who is normally the Rock of Gibraltar for everyone. Stress and not feeling good can result in some extreme emotional mood swings and blow ups that lead to actual arguments. The important thing Cancer Warriors, and Companion Caregivers as well, if you find yourselves frustrated, irritated… dare I say, pissed off? If a situation arises where the argument seems insurmountable, is stubborn and ongoing during the course of cancer treatment, stop and remind each other why you

are there with each other. The Companion Care giver is
there because the Cancer Warrior cared about them and
asked them to be there, they came because they cared.
After working out the real issue and making up, then you
can have a good laugh together about how really close you
came to using the "I've Got Cancer Card".

   I remember one day, near the end of treatments I was
being quite stubborn, and insisting I was not going for my
radiation treatment that day. I felt that I could miss one
treatment. Plenty of other people were missing
appointments. We heard conversations about that very
topic almost every day. My face was so swollen from the
chemo treatment the day before and I complained my mask
would not fit, it was so cold out, and I was nauseous; I
really just did not feel good at all and did not want to go. I
had plenty of good excuses in other words. I was really
feeling quite spectacularly splendidly obstinate and ornery
that day. My oldest daughter Tennille was with me that
week, and she was quite the little drill sergeant let me tell
you. With eight years as a Marine under her belt, I really
mean this literally. She would wake me to be sure I took my
nausea medications on a strict time schedule, and would
push fluids to maintain hydration (Trying to sneak water in
through the PEG tube was T's idea), she would insist on
eating when it was time to eat and she certainly was not
letting me miss an appointment. I had not missed one
single appointment, I even had to go for a radiation
treatment on Christmas Eve, and she had decided I sure as
heck was not missing one on her watch. I was really in a
bad, bad, ready to put my foot down, I'm missing this
appointment no matter what, mood that day, let me tell
you. We exchanged words back and forth for some time,
and it really did get quite heated. How dare this young
Whipper Snapper think she could make me, her mother, do

anything I didn't want to? We were getting closer and closer to time to leave. Then she threatened to pick me up and carry me out to the car. Dead silence; as dead silent as she was dead serious. Then she said very calmly "It won't be pretty, because I'm not as big as Kevin, but you will be in that car". Her little face was so set, so determined, so serious…. such a Marine. Mine was set too though, dark and stubborn. We locked eyes and it was at that moment I saw she meant what she said, I really was going, but I also saw that there was no anger there, only love and concern. Like a refreshing cool rain, sanity washed over me banishing my anger. Like the sun breaking through a bank of thunderous storm clouds I started laughing. I was laughing because the picture that came to my mind was of the two of us physically scrapping and rolling on the ground. Even at the lowest point of treatment inside I was still the tough athletic scrapper, and Tennille was right, it would not have been pretty. It was the graphic picture in my mind that really brought it home for me. I didn't want to fight with Tennille. That would be crazy, I love T. At first when I started laughing I think she really thought I had lost it. I told her about my mental image and we were both caught up laughing together and embellishing upon our imaginary blow by blow battle as we wrestled and crashed through the house. Between gasps of laughter I gathered my stuff for the trip, conceding victory, and with a chuckle and a smile started urging her to hurry up if we were going before I changed my mind. It had been an exciting morning to say the least; releasing emotions, good or bad, can be exhausting. As we made slow careful progress from the porch out to the car, I was leaning against her for support and wisenheimer Tennille says, in a funny mafia guy voice, "Okay time to stuff you in the car." Fresh gales of laughter hit us and I was so weak and laughing so uncontrollably about how hard it would have been to stuff me in the car that she *kind of did* have to stuff me in the car.

BEFORE THE NEXT ANGRY WORD IN A SERIOUS SITUATION LOOK EACH OTHER IN THE EYES AND REMIND EACH OTHER WHY YOU'RE THERE.

I mention these tips for dealing with emotional outbursts and arguments only because I know they really can happen, I have seen them occur quite often. Sometimes the silliest of little disagreements or comments can unleash an unexpected flood of tears or a torrent of angry words. I have seen arguments erupt about almost anything you can think of; from misunderstandings over financial arrangements and bills, to he said she said situations regarding gossip conversations… I mean once I saw an argument about putting things in the refrigerator in the wrong place (God Bless you Janie). Why do we snap and lash out? Because going through cancer treatments that can last for months at a time wears down everyone involved. Often the cancer patient is so weak that the only things left that are in their control anymore are what they can reach out and touch and see around them and they can get picky, for example about where things are put or what the temperature of the home is set at. Fear of the unknown and the uncertainty of the outcome can get to the best of us, even the most patient saint like people sometimes. It happens. What is important is that we work through and forgive.

DO NOT CUT STRONG TIES WITH A FAMILY MEMBER OR FRIEND IN THE MIDST OF CANCER TREATMENTS OVER A BLOW UP,

PLAY THE CANCER CARD, DO WHAT YOU MUST, BUT MAKE UP.

I think that is important to share this little bit about arguing because I worry that some may not think it can happen, and I know many may read this and shake their heads, thinking well that is crazy "we never argue at all so of course we will not argue while battling cancer". Trust me, it happens. There is a lot of thought and mental activity and raw emotions going on while a person is going through cancer treatments; a lot of what ifs and I wishes and never got to… the deeper we progress into an especially rigorous cancer treatment course the worse, the weaker, the less sure about making it we can become. Nearing the end of treatments, by the time you are reaching that last two weeks and counting mark you might be feeling like I just can't do it. You might start thinking I'm not going to make it. You may even start irritating/scaring your companion caregivers by beginning conversations out of the blue with "I wanted you to know, just in case I die…" Listen to me and remember this;

THE LAST FEW WEEKS OF CANCER TREATMENTS ARE THE HARDEST AND MAY EVEN HAVE YOU THINKING THOUGHTS THAT YOU'RE NOT GOING TO MAKE IT, I KNOW BECAUSE I DID… AND I'M STILL HERE. DO NOT GIVE IN.

I remember periods of being that quiet person that didn't bother joining in on conversations sometimes. Granted in my case I had trouble speaking of course with throat cancer. I was often just lost in much deeper thoughts than the weather, or what was for dinner, or who was getting what for Christmas. I was busy thinking about things I wished I had done and things I wished I had not, things I wished were different. I did not "withdraw" from everyone, I was just quieter and more retrospective, often pondering simple pleasures in life that maybe I used to just take for granted. Sometimes I would just be imagining being in a happy place. One of my favorites was a grassy spot on the sunny side of a quiet lake, and I would enjoy the breeze and watching the clouds changing into shapes over head. Normal innocent conversations about things going on in daily life would sometimes become background noise. I even scared my husband one day when I decided I needed to have an "If I die" conversation. Poor man I told him that no matter what he had to buy that last plot by Mom, Dad and Larry for me. I guess my advice to the cancer warriors would be don't panic if you start experiencing these "deep" thoughts, you're not alone; it's only human to wonder and worry, especially when we are at particularly weak and vulnerable points in our lives.

CANCER WARRIORS IT'S OKAY TO PONDER THE GREAT MYSTERIES OF LIFE BUT DON'T LET YOUR DOMINATING THOUGHTS BE MORBID ONES.

To the caregiver/companions, who we may occasionally scare the crap out of with what seem to be morbid thoughts, I would say, Humor us. My husband's first response to hearing my burial wishes was "Well you're not going to die so it doesn't matter". To me it did matter though. This led into a major and altogether unnecessarily exhausting discussion (argument), until he finally agreed if anything happened he would make sure my brothers helped with arrangements. Needless to say he was right... I did not need the plot.

COMPANION CAREGIVERS IT IS OKAY TO SAY THINGS LIKE DON'T BE SILLY YOU ARE NOT GOING TO DIE, BUT FIRST REMEMBER TO SAY "I HEAR YOU, AND I WILL REMEMBER WHAT YOU SAID."

So here we are the last day of treatment. As a part of the final goodbyes and well wishes that took place in the radiation treatment room and extended out into the lobby waiting area before I left after my last treatment I was also given my plastic mesh radiation treatment restraint mask to take with me. What a morbid memento if you ask me, and I said as much. I didn't want it; I had hated being locked into place under that thing every day. The techs said that most people took theirs though. I said "I don't want it". I was too tired to really care if I brought that thing home, quite frankly by my last day of treatment I probably was not a good person to ask to make any decisions. I was pretty miserable and I admit it, often quite grumpy even though I tried not to be. Kevin was worried I might want it later though and insisted we bring it. I wouldn't carry it on my lap, I left him to manage it and the wheelchair, and after stopping at the desk to schedule follow up appointments he wheeled me out to the car for the last time from the bat cave.

Other survivors I have spoken with since that day have told me they gained satisfaction destroying their radiation masks by various nefarious means. These ranged from imaginative forms of burning and melting to running over with cars, and even using it for a tug of war match with their dog as a chew toy (I wouldn't recommend the last one…not sure if it would be a good idea in case Fido swallowed any of it). It came home with us and it was quite some time before I even thought of it again. Eventually after consideration instead of going up in a brief flaming revolt against the uncompromising restraint it had come to symbolize, the pale yellow radiation mask retired to the closet where it sat until I got it out briefly to take a photo for the cover of this book. For me it is a silent reminder of struggle and perseverance, of hopelessness and hope. After undergoing radiation treatments if you had a restraint mask, or similar body part restraint mold your first reaction may be the same as mine was, I don't want it, I hate that thing.

IF YOUR RADIATION TREATMENT MASK/MOLD IS OFFERED AS A MEMENTO, BRING IT HOME, YOU CAN ALWAYS DECIDE WHAT TO DO WITH IT LATER WHEN YOU DO NOT HATE THE SITE OF IT SO MUCH. IF IT IS NOT OFFERED YOU COULD ASK FOR IT IF YOU LIKE.

There is one last thing you need to do on the day of your very last scheduled cancer treatment…

MARK THE DATE TREATMENT ENDS ON YOUR CALENDAR BECAUSE EVERY YEAR FROM THAT DAY FORWARD THIS IS YOUR NEW AFTER CANCER BIRTHDAY.

Section II *Life During Cancer* has covered diagnosis, staging, treatment options and tips on how to survive them, and now that the very last scheduled treatment is completed it is time to move on to Section III *Life Beyond Cancer*, which can be easier to read about than to do. *This is why* Chapter 9, *Cut Loose*, intentionally begins with a slight overlap back to this final chapter of *Life With Cancer;* it is about a fragile transition period fraught with unexpected surprises that is often the last barrier to be overcome between being a cancer patient who has survived cancer treatments and acknowledging and accepting the new title of being a Survivor.

Your Footsteps May Not Be Quite As Firm As They Were Coming Into Section II Life With Cancer, But You Are Still Here And Now It Is Time To Take The First Shaky Steps Into Life Beyond Cancer...

SECTION III: LIFE BEYOND CANCER
9 LIFE BEYOND CANCER
CUT LOOSE

Cut Loose offers insight and advice about a very specific window of time; the immediate post treatment period. Some may think "Isn't this the easy Part?" "Isn't the day after all those cancer treatments are finished a time for celebration and happiness"? For the companion caregivers it certainly can be, but often for the Cancer Warrior these expected happy reactions tend to be very subdued and can be delayed for quite some time. There are a number of reasons for this and this chapter will address some of these immediate post treatment issues and concerns that are often unexpected but unfortunately frequently encountered during those early limbo like weeks of *Life Beyond Cancer*. This very personal and pivotal immediate post treatment blues/slump period seems to be a little over looked or under rated in available literature. At least to me it did.

The day my treatments ended no one said to me "Okay you're a cancer survivor go forth and live again". They slid me out on the treatment table from inside that MRI like tunnel that had delivered those invisible beams of radiation every day, for two months and somehow shrunk my tumor to almost nothing, just like they did on every other day. The only difference was that day when they unlocked my very much disliked by that point restraint mask for the last time, CLICK! CLICK! CLICK! CLICK! CLICK! 5 final Clicks to freedom, there was a very festive air in the room.

All the techs were smiling and telling me "congratulations you're done with treatments" and there were a lot of well wishes and "Good Luck", hugs all around from nurses and technicians, even doctors from different departments that I did not know. The atmosphere almost felt like I should be seeing streamers of confetti and a grand launch of colorful balloons any minute. Was I getting on a ship and everyone waving Bon Voyage as I set out? Strangely enough, looking back now I realize that it was the start of a new journey; new routines, new worries and new challenges, I just didn't realize it at the time. I was no longer a cancer patient actively battling cancer, because treatments were completed. What or who was I then?

A MENTAL TRANSFORMATION NEEDS TO TAKE PLACE, A TIME OF LETTING GO OF BEING A CANCER PATIENT AND EMBRACING BECOMING A CANCER SURVIVOR AND IT CAN BE A VERY SLOW AND DIFFICULT PROCESS.

There was the expected general advice of course like "take care of myself", and "don't forget to stay hydrated", and after a last parting reminder "do not hesitate to call my doctor if I needed anything" Debra had left the building. The only thing missing from the celebration, as far as I was concerned, was someone actually saying "Okay you are cured there is no more cancer". No one said that, because they all knew that it would months before actually learning if the cancer had been defeated or not.

All along as treatments progressed my doctors kept me updated, as most oncology teams will, especially when asked. They did tell me after the third or fourth week that they felt the tumor was beginning to respond to treatment. After that point they continued to assure me "things are looking good" and encouraged me to hang in there. At each of the radiation treatments while I was in the machine they were able to visualize the tumor, and at each meeting with my doctors I was given the good news that "The tumor had been shrinking steadily". They were also pleased with progress regarding the nearby lymph nodes that were being targeted as well, because they were possible cancer storage units of a sort. By the last week of treatments I was told they could no longer actually see the tumor. This was really a bit misleading though. Was the cancer gone? They did not say that, only that they could no longer visualize the tumor.

They were not saying they were sure the tumor was *Gone*, because they did not know, it just couldn't be seen anymore. That was because by this point, after 36 rounds of radiation treatments, everything was just so inflamed, there was so much edema (swelling), and dead tissue that quite frankly I don't think any of the structures of my throat were quite recognizable by then. So they could not see the tumor, but it was not possible yet to know for sure if it was all the way gone or just very small, hidden, and waiting to grow back.

IT IS QUITE COMMON THAT AT THE TIME TREATMENTS OFFICIALLY END IT IS NOT POSSIBLE TO DETERMINE WHETHER THE CANCER IS GONE OR NOT.

A cancer survivor sometimes has a very lengthy wait

ahead of them before the sweet victory of the words "You are cancer free" will be heard. That first "day after" I felt like a balloon freed from its string and I wasn't sure where I was going to float to. The aggressive cancer treatment regime which from day of diagnosis to last treatment had consumed my life from October 13th 2009 – January 21st 2010, I'm not going to lie I was so exhausted that there was no rejoicing energy in me. and recovery seemed a very distant dream at that point.

Depending on how rigorous and lengthy the treatment cycles have been there are many cancer warriors who will feel like reaching that final treatment day has just about drained all of the inner resources they had to call upon. Any one undergoing radiation treatments for Head/neck or throat cancers may encounter the challenges and pain of oral and throat tissue deterioration and compromised salivary gland function, and some strong chemotherapy treatments will have a similar effect as well. While this condition became quite painful before the end of the long term treatment plan was reached, tissues will continue to deteriorate and often pain actually becomes even worse after the official end of treatments. It did for me.

MANY CANCER WARRIORS ACTUALLY TAKE A TURN FOR THE WORSE IN THE POST TREATMENT PERIOD INITIALLY, BOTH PHYSICALLY AND EMOTIONALLY, BEFORE ROUNDING THE BEND TOWARDS RECOVERY.

Information and advice pertaining to the post treatment recovery period which is overlapping and beyond this Immediate post treatment adjustment period will be discussed in greater detail within chapter 10 *Reaching a point of Feeling Better and Staying There*, for now it is important to note that as mentioned earlier;

RADIATION TREATMENTS CAN CONTINUE TO DO THEIR WORK AND "COOK" FOR A NUMBER OF WEEKS AFTER ACTUAL TREATMENTS END.

Most of this so far is not exactly the news you want to hear after making it through the treatments, but it is information worth having. Knowing in advance about these very real physical and mental challenges that can combine and affect the health of cancer survivors in the immediate post treatment period, raising awareness in advance that for a time after treatments end there may actually be a continued deterioration in health and attitude can make a difference.

Not knowing whether the cancer was gone like I said was one of the biggest immediate road blocks to charging forward into *Life Beyond Cancer* for me, ranking right up there next to the fact that I felt closer to dying than I had at any point in my treatments. Of course the doctors will keep you updated on progress all through the course of the treatments, they share with you whether or not they feel the treatment plan seems to be *working*, but on the day most patients are *Cut Loose* from the daily treatment routine no one will say "you are cured the cancer is gone". This news at the end of treatments comes as a major shock to many of us; "wait a minute, we survived the battle, made it through treatments, but the war is not over yet"? This is one of the reasons that the time of "celebration" and "joy", the "relief" that was so deserved and expected after treatments end is often missing. I think not knowing this in advance could actually have an almost boomerang effect on mental health for the cancer patient trying to transform into the cancer survivor that they truly are. I felt like I did not even get to breathe a sigh of relief before I was holding my breath in fear again. You won that battle against the treatments, and it was a hard fought one too most likely, so take the advice from someone who knows, do not short change yourself like I did at first, own it, and embrace it, you made it through treatments.

YOU ARE A SURVIVOR YOU SURVIVED TREATMENTS AND AT THIS WEAKEST POINT LET NO ONE TAKE THAT ACHIEVEMENT AWAY FROM YOU.

So after going through weeks that turned into months, now we wait weeks, which can actually be more like months, before finding out if the cancer is really gone? This is unfortunately what happens in many cases. I actually had to wait six long months before my first post treatment PET scan to find out if my doctors felt the cancer was really gone. Yes you read that right, six months. This delay is because the treatment target area needs recovery time for tissues to heal and things to kind of fall back into place after all the swelling and trauma. Also the area is usually what they call "hot", and this can make it difficult to accurately visualize the sugar based tracer used in PET scans. That is also why sometimes insurance company policies can cause a delay too, they do not want false positives. They tend to be a bit stingy with the PET scans IMHO. Blood work and lab results will continue to be monitored for clues or warning signs throughout this time, but the PET scan is what most are waiting for after the end of treatments because it is generally considered the gold standard for "cancer Free" status. It was a long half of a year in which I should have spent the entire time focused on recovery and being positive, instead of a portion of it allowing doubts and worries and negative thoughts to fester.

I think it might have been helpful easing through the transition period if I had understood better in advance that they would not know for so long after treatments ended whether or not the cancer was actually gone. To be honest I had been thinking they wouldn't know right away, especially since I was aware of possible metastases concerns post treatment from my own research as well as experiences of fellow patients. It was just that when the doctors were saying they could not see it anymore at all… well I guess I just let myself get a little overly hopeful. The higher you get the further you fall sometimes. When it was explained they were not saying the cancer was gone, they were just saying they couldn't see it anymore it really bummed me out major. I think if I had understood in advance that the cancer treatments themselves were one step to get through, and that there would be a lengthy pause before the next step, to determine success or failure, I may have taken it in stride better than I did.

YOUR DOCTORS, YOUR CASE, AND YOUR EXPERIENCE ARE INDIVIDUAL; THIS WILL DETERMINE WAIT TIME FOR A DEFINITE PROGNOSIS. I KNOW IT SOUNDS CLICHÉ' BUT THINK POSITIVE EITHER WAY!

Like I said I wasted a lot of time and energy worrying about whether the treatments killed the cancer or not and about whether or not the PET scan when I did have it would reveal a new cancer, a metastasis to a new site. This possibility was especially concerning to me because I had been told from the start of treating my Stage IVB cancer that if this plan of action failed there would be no additional treatment choices left for me. Make sure you to talk to your oncologists; this is certainly **not** true in all cases, especially if you have a cancer that was caught early. The problem was I had already received the maximum dosage of radiation treatments allowed, and my chemo doctor had also said the same about my Big Guns chemotherapy treatment… if it did not work there was no backup plan because it was the strongest chemo agent available. People can, have and often do receive treatments for additional cancers, but in most cases it is usually after time has passed. I think what they meant was more along the lines of if this didn't work my body wouldn't be up to surviving any additional treatments. Given the shape I was in at the end of treatments, they were right.

We cannot let ourselves become focused on whether the cancer is "gone" or whether there will be metastasis to other locations, it really is a waste of time and you can worry yourself sick for nothing. Trust me. I had to wait, yes, but after worrying and waiting for that first one, it was worth it, it was clean. Subsequent yearly PET scans have been likewise. I worried for nothing. I know it is really hard to just say "Oh all right Deb said don't worry in between end of treatments and waiting for that first PET scan so I won't". I know you will worry, but try not to let it be your main concern, you will have plenty of time to worry later, right now is a time to focus on rest, taking good care of yourself and regaining strength.

I wish I could get back some of that time I spent being angry, or pouting I guess would be a better word in those immediate weeks after treatment ended. It took me a little while to shake myself out of the mentally negative slump I had let myself get into and put my focus back where it

belonged, on what was now instead of what if later. I had
to give myself a pep talk. I had to figure all these things out
for myself and it took a while. It took me by surprise when
I thought the cancer was gone and then learned maybe not.
It took me by surprise when I learned how long I would
have to wait until I could find out if the cancer was really
gone, at least knowing in advance you can talk to your
doctor about this before treatments end. If you do find out
that you will have to wait for a lengthy period of time
before finding out if the cancer is gone at least the news
will not take you completely by surprise and bum you out
right at the end of treatments.

IN THIS CRUCIAL POST TREATMENT PERIOD NO SURPRISES ARE GOOD SURPRISES.

There was one more aspect of ending treatments that
was really a surprise; the void that was left in the wake of
finishing treatments. It seemed like there was such a
complete vacuum when the daily routine of treatment
ended so abruptly. One day there was all this purpose, I
was getting up for a reason, I was fighting cancer. I went to
appointments every day and I was in a medical setting and
around medical professionals, doctors and nurses, able to
talk to them on a daily basis about any concerns. I had so
whole heartedly adjusted to the routine when I entered
treatment, so focused on the start and making it through,
that I never really thought about the day I would finish. By
the time I was half way through treatments I wasn't really
thinking or planning ahead for much of anything except
doing the same thing the next day quite frankly. I didn't
realize the treatment period would be so intense, or how
bad I would feel by the time they ended, or how abrupt the
end of treatments would seem.

Fighting cancer was my normal, being around the medical facility and seeing doctors every day was my normal. Have you ever heard of Stockholm syndrome? Usually it is used in discussion about kidnapping victims becoming dependant and/or attached to their captors? It was like the cancer and the treatments had been holding me captive. My days had revolved around it. I had become comfortable with fighting cancer and even though I didn't realize it at the time there must have been some sense of security gained being around the medical setting and professionals daily. There had also been a camaraderie developed with other cancer patients in various stages of treatment that I felt was lost too abruptly as well in many cases, because we would no longer be seeing the doctor on the same day of the week if they were still in treatment or finished sooner. Again I remind friends you make in waiting areas for cancer treatment, exchange contact information, that is why you have that smaller contacts pad. Not being "family" it is not uncommon to make a friend in treatment, for example meeting in the chemo lounge over an eight hour day infusion session, or in one of the waiting areas on a daily basis, and then due to changes in schedules you lose touch. Each of you left wondering how each other is doing with no way to inquire without that personal contact information. Instead of being glad treatments had ended, at first I felt a weird sense of loss and almost abandonment. I felt like "I'm not ready to be on my own yet, I'm not cured I want to still be a cancer patient." I had Stockholm syndrome.

I realized I was feeling crabby and negative because in some strange way I was missing the normal, the security, of the treatment routine. Even though I did not completely understand these feelings, by talking with others after those first few weeks post treatment I understood enough to know it was real and more common than thought. I was missing the treatments I had come to hate so much. I knew I needed to shake off my heebie jeebies, let myself get comfortable with being a survivor and just relax, and rest, enjoy a little sunshine and hope instead of doom and gloom for a while. It wasn't easy to let go of being a "patient" and becoming a survivor. State of Mind just like during diagnosis is important and I needed to put mine in the right place.

THE END OF TREATMENTS CAN UNLEASH AN UNEXPECTED FLOOD OF EMOTIONS; YOU MAY FIND INSECURITY AND FEAR IN A NECK AND NECK RACE WITH ANGER AND DISAPPOINTMENT.

Keep your family and friends support system close by. Maintain, establish or resume Communications with fellow survivors, people you exchanged contact information with, either via phone or online through one of the recommended forums or one of many others that are available.

DO NOT THINK YOU HAVE TO HESITATE AT ALL IF YOU FEEL YOU NEED TO SEE ONE OF YOUR DOCTORS, KNOW THEY WILL FIT YOU IN IF YOU SAY YOU NEED THEM.

I had found myself absolutely, completely, physically and emotionally used up, at my weakest, weighing all of about 86 pounds and in the most pain than I had been in up to this point through all of the treatments, when I was "cut loose" on a Monday. My treatments had been supposed to end on a Friday in the outlook planned, but I think it was the New Year's holiday that bumped it into the beginning of the next week at some point for my last radiation treatment. So my last treatment day was on a Monday. Monday was a very busy day in the office with more new patients coming in than patients checking out of treatment. Making the follow up appointments at the reception desk turned into a drawn out and complicated affair. All three doctors wanted to see me the "Next week" they had said, but each department had their own schedules which would be different days from treatment schedules, and none saw post treatment patients on the same day apparently. The chemotherapy doctor who I used to see on Tuesdays would now want to see me on Thursday mornings, but I would need to come in at least one to two days before appointments to have blood drawn in the lab so he could have the results when I did see him. The ENT Oncologists had a surgery schedule and new patient intake day to work around and it was looking like possibly Wednesdays for him, and I could go to the lab and get the blood work drawn for the chemo doctor the day I was in to see him. In Radiation Oncology I couldn't do my usual once a week meeting with the doctor on Thursdays like I used to, because that was when he had weekly appointments with patients "in treatment", like I used to be. Details, details, Mondays and Wednesdays were new patient in take days, people getting masks made and the initial welcome to treatments tour, and I was just kind of listening to it all like blah blah blah, in one ear and out the other at that point, thinking in my head "Just give me a print out of the schedule so I can go". After all of the finger tapping on the keyboard my initial follow up appointment for the radiation doctor, who I was supposed to see first post treatment, since it was a Monday, and he had scribbled "next week" in the follow up directions (he was probably thinking it was Thursday the day I usually saw him), worked out to be all the way to the next Friday. Almost a full two weeks. That did worry me, and seemed like a long time, but I didn't say anything, I was tired and just wanted to be home and done. Kevin voiced my thoughts though; waving the radiation mask he was carrying in the direction of my slight blanket wrapped form slumped in the wheelchair beside him, "Two Weeks… in this condition?" She said she could "try" to fit me in, but to me, in my tired crabby mind that translated to another twenty minutes of finger tapping on a keyboard with the result being I would wait extra long on the day of the appointment because I was "fit in". It was an effort to speak up, but I managed to rasp out in my scratchy, heavy breathing gravelly voice "just take the Friday appointment I want to go home, if we need to we can call".

BE SURE THE RECEPTIONISTS UNDERSTAND YOUR DOCTOR'S INTENTIONS WHEN MAKING THOSE FIRST FOLLOW UP APPOINTMENTS TO AVOID MISUNDERSTANDING; DO NOT BE GRUMPY AND STUBBORN LIKE I WAS.

We did know the doctor did not intend to wait so long to see me back, because he was concerned over my condition, but in his notes for follow up he had written "next week" and the receptionist took that literally. Quite frankly I was just too grumpy, had waited long enough and wanted out the door with the ride home done and to be home in my bed to want to bother trying to go through changing one appointment, which would have changed all of the others.

I must say in my defense here that I had grown very touchy and irritable about "waiting" times as my treatments had progressed, and by the end I really had no patience for hold ups and waiting at all. There is a lot of "waiting" involved. I tried not to be so grumpy, I kept my irritation for the most part just festering in my mind, and outwardly acted like everything was fine, on most days. I really did try to be a patient (adjective) patient (Noun) but it was just such an effort to stay in an upright sitting position for extended periods of time. This was especially true by the end of treatments; my neck had become very weak and painful to the point I could barley hold up and balance my own head. I understood most of the time the waiting was because I had good doctors who spent time talking to their patients. It made sense of course as treatments progressed and the condition of a patient worsened the more time they would want to talk to their doctor. The day my radiation oncology doctor followed me in through that emergency room admission and started the IV line that no one else was able to get in for me, he left patients waiting for quite a while I am sure. This advice was something I had to work very hard to keep in mind then, as well as going to my first post follow up appointments. It is very common for doctors to run a bit behind schedule when seeing patients towards the end of treatment and during those first couple of months into recovery. This wasn't a doctor though it was a receptionist, and I let it be known I wanted to go.

I did not want to wait anymore or think, or worry whether the cancer was gone or not, or if it would pop back up as a metastatic cancer somewhere else, all I wanted at that moment was to go home and curl up somewhere quiet like a feral animal and lick my wounds in peace. I had no thoughts or plans for what I was going to do as a cancer survivor that day because as far as I was concerned I wasn't even a cancer survivor yet. No one had told me I was. For me, for a while that long awaited day treatments ended was just the beginning of a new, cruel, very frightening, and frustrating waiting game.

Would additional post treatment support be a good idea? Perhaps, but a better understanding in advance of what this immediate post treatment period is like can ease many of the negative thoughts and worries somewhat. A continued physical decline may not be as frightening if expected, and understanding the end of treatments is not really an end of cancer is an aspect we should all know about. It is a cancer recovery aspect that is gaining a little more attention recently I think. Perhaps when recounting cancer experiences we want to convey a more positive and encouraging outlook and tend to avoid talking about the parts we experienced that we did not understand, or that we think may be discouraging because it was an area we feel we failed in? We do not like to admit we were afraid or doubted ourselves sometimes. I only know I had no one telling me to expect these things in advance, I experienced them as I went through them.

I noticed even the forums tended to be rather quiet on this phase. I myself fell silent for a while online. For me, as far as activity on the forums, I kind of had a "if I didn't have anything good to say, I wasn't saying anything at all" attitude. I didn't want to discourage people nearing the end of their treatments by complaining what it was like when they were done with them. Once back into scheduled appointments forum input tends to pick back up again with updates on what the doctors are saying, and discussion about how we feel at that point now that we have decided we are going to survive, and everyone forgets that scary disappointing time frame that follows immediately after cancer treatments end.

I had to push my weary broken body and mind along and stumbled blindly through the no man's land of that immediate post treatment slump, doom and gloom, like many others before and many who will come after. Chapter 9 focused on emotional pitfalls and unwanted surprises encountered in the immediate post treatment period, which hopefully with this knowledge will be a brief(er), now it is all about moving onward and upward to Chapter 10, *Rounding The Bend* which begins the day after the end of treatments and continues two years into the future.

10 ROUNDING THE BEND

Whether it takes us a few days or weeks to mentally decide to be survivors and get back into our stride we need to take care of our weakened and fragile physical body to the best of our ability as we move from completing treatments to completing recovery. Here again there is an intentional overlapping time frame between Chapters, with healthcare tips and advice in *Rounding The Bend* beginning from the low point of the day after cancer treatments end, the recuperation period, to the high point of that first clean PET scan when survivors will finally be granted full-fledged Cancer free Survivor status by those in the medical profession, and beyond to the two year maximum recovery mark, an important step in the timeline of cancer survivors.

On the first day post cancer treatments hopefully forewarned with the knowledge from chapter 9 *Cut Loose* you are not spending it being pissy and grumpy because there were too many surprises the day before. You knew in advance to speak frankly with your doctor before treatments ended about these surprises and you knew there would not be an immediate prognosis post treatment. You may have been bummed out at learning how long the wait will be before knowing for sure if the treatments were successful or not, but it did not come as a surprise at the end of treatments, you expected this wait. You are also not feeling quite so cut loose and left in the lurch because you are ready for the change in routine, and you have also made sure that your first follow up appointments are within a comfortable and safe span of time, and not two weeks away. By the way my radiation doctor actually called my house that next Wednesday looking for me, asking where I had been and how I was. He was mad because he knew that I knew darn well he wanted to see me in 4-5 days, not a whole two weeks away. I hope everyone has at least one doctor on their team like Dr. B. was for me. Seriously, if he thinks you need to be admitted in the middle of winter when he sees you for your weekly appointment with him, he will hide your shoes to try to keep you from leaving.

INSTEAD OF STRESSING OVER CHANGES IN ROUTINES, YOU WILL BEGIN MAKING NEW ONES, UNIQUE AND ADAPTED TO YOUR SITUATION.

Instead of being hit with a bunch of these last minute surprises you were prepared and instead of worrying over future what if and maybe's you are ready to concentrate on right now, on strengthening and healing; finding the path that will take you around this bend in the road and on the straight and narrow to recovery.

So with no appointments what exactly do we do with that first day, and the day after that, and the next and the next? For starters go easy on yourself, but at the same time don't go completely soft. At this stage of recovery it is very tempting to just make use of pain medication if cancer treatments have left you with pain that is being managed, as is often the case, and curl up all comfy cozy in bed, wrapped in blankets, surrounded with pillows, flipping through TV stations and having companion/caregivers wait on us hand and foot. This option is even more tempting if cancer treatments end during cold weather winter months, like January when it is freezing outside. Rest really is first and foremost a very important part of recovery, and you definitely do not want to be over exerting or taxing yourself at this early stage. For that first day you really can go ahead and just relax, you deserve it, but be sure to read on because there is more that must be done besides sleep and rest while recuperating.

ADEQUATE SLEEP AND REST IS CRUCIAL DURING RECOVERY BECAUSE AS NOTED EARLIER CELL REGENERATION IS AT OPTIMUM PERFORMANCE DURING DEEP SLEEP.

You will find in the early stages of recovery, what I consider a recuperation period, that much of the advice offered in *Keeping A Light On At The End Of The Tunnel* is still solid gold, so forgive if some of this sounds redundant or repetitious but many of these tips from that Old Routine will still be very beneficial and many do not realize how important it is that some of them are continued into the post treatment recovery period for quite a while. This period of recovery, or getting around the bend, varies greatly from one individual to the next, as has been discussed previously. For example cancers detected very early may not need to be treated so aggressively as later stage or larger cancers, and blood cancers such as Leukemia may go into remission and show rapid drastic improvement or conversely take a turn for the worse and have a rapid worsening of symptoms. Each treatment and recovery cycle is individual.

I can give you an idea how long initial "recuperation" may take, based upon the point that "I" actually started to feel like I was really coming around the bend and felt I was continuing to steadily improve. I am not saying feeling great, but to a point I knew I was steadily improving at least. I can also tell you that my opinion and my doctors differed greatly on this point. My ENT doctor was very slow and reluctant to voice optimism and declare me a post treatment survivor "on the way" to recovery. His opinion happened to be a very important one though. Remember the PEG tube I had? The whole story about this will be revealed later, and hopefully give you a shocked chuckle at my expense, but for now let me just say that it was up to my ENT to decide when I would not need it anymore and by Mid April that PEG tube was still with me. My ENT said he would not remove it until he had seen a marked improvement happening in my throat instead of further deterioration. So how long until you really feel like you are starting to get better? Between my opinion and that of my doctors 3-4 months of recuperation had passed before I "rounded the bend" and made the turn onto the road to recovery. Again I am not saying I was feeling great by the third month, but at least I felt like I was getting a little stronger as the days passed beyond that point. I remind again here radiation treatments continue to work for some time beyond last treatment, and an overall deterioration in general health and well being can and usually does continue for a few weeks after the end of treatments. That is why it is so important that some of the routines from treatment follow into the recovery period.

CONTINUE TO MOISTURIZE SKIN WITH PRESCRIBED CREAM OR DOCTOR APPROVED ALOE OR SIMILAR LOTION WITHIN RADIATION TARGET AREA A MINIMUM OF 2X PER DAY.

If you have experienced detrimental affects to the oral cavity and/or throat it is absolutely 100% imperative that extra care and attention to the oral environment continues uninterrupted. Individuals who have undergone radiation cancer treatment for head/neck or throat cancer and/or chemo cycles which involved the use of exceptionally strong chemotherapy agents for any cancer, it is very likely this overall condition will worsen further before it actually begins to improve. It may sound gross but dead and dying tissue from within the target area will continue to slough off for some time. The saliva that is produced may be very thick at this time, and it may be even more difficult to keep your throat clear of it. The thick ropy strands of saliva may require clearing more often.

The dry mouth aspect may become more of a pronounced problem during this time and better attention to oral care now will improve future overall outcome. At first, with so many other things going on in the post cancer treatment recovery period, aches and pains, appointments and weariness, all vying for your attention, the dry mouth may not have even been bad enough yet that you realized yet how really dry your mouth has been. The condition can sneak up over time, and you may have even gotten kind of used to it as salivary production decreased slowly over the course of treatments and beyond due to damaged salivary glands. This collateral damage may result in long term and even lifetime dry mouth or xerostomia. The important thing to remember is the healing process will be helped along with continued frequent gargling, rinsing and attention to detail on proper oral care. I cannot stress the importance of this enough. There will be a battle in the future to protect and maintain the health of your teeth, they will not only be in danger from the effects of a dry mouth environment but may also be weakened by the cancer treatments as well, especially in the case of head/neck and throat cancers. The time to actively start aggressive maintenance dental care is here and now.

A) EVERY EFFORT SHOULD BE MADE TO MAINTAIN ADEQUATE LEVELS OF MOISTURE IN THE ORAL CAVITY AS THIS ENCOURAGES HEALING OF SORES AND MINIMIZES FORMATION OF NEW ONES. STAY HYDRATED.

B) BE SURE TO RENEW PRESCRIPTION FOR THE MAGIC MOUTHWASH OR SIMILAR RINSE OF CHOICE, BESIDES NUMBING BENEFIT IT SHOULD BE MILDLY ANTI BACTERIAL, CONTINUE FREQUENT RINSING AND GARGLING.

C) ONCE A DAY BAKING SODA RINSES ARE HELPFUL FOR MAINTAINING PROPER PH BALANCE AS WELL.

Feel free to take it easy as you move through the recuperation process. Curling up flipping channels wrapped in a blanket like I said works great in moderation, but I would recommend at first to at least continue with the stretching and deep breathing exercises, especially the deep breathing. No matter how low we are feeling we need to move around. The last thing that you want to do after everything you have been through is to lay down flat out for three or four days straight and risk developing pneumonia or blood clots from not moving. Rest is good but in proper moderation like everything else. Remaining immobile for longer than a normal 8 hour night of sleep is not good for you. I'm not going to highlight the exercise points here and push you to over exert yourself, I leave that up to you to know what you feel able to do and when you feel able to do it, as long as you do it.

EVEN ON THE DAYS YOU ARE TAKING IT EASY IF ABLE MAKE YOURSELF GET UP AND WALK AROUND FOR BRIEF PERIODS EVERY FEW HOURS.

My daughter Tennille made a very good point that motivated me on the morning of the third day "You know if you were not laying there in bed because we were done with treatments right about now we would be making our way down to the bat cave from the top of the parking garage". She made me realize she was right; not only that I should try to be moving around more, but that I should be glad I wasn't being forced to endure going outside in the cold morning everyday anymore. Just thinking about the cold and the drive up there and getting in and out for appointments and the drive home again made me really realize/think/appreciate at that moment how much easier I had it when I made the mental comparison between doing that and getting up and shuffling around a bit more in the warm cozy house. I guess I'm just saying try to stay as mobile and motivated as you are able. You do not want to let yourself turn into a tin man, because we humans do not have any magical oil cans that will get us moving again.

It is also very important to try to avoid coming down with things like simple colds and flues. Try to limit contact with people known to have a bug or cold while still in a fragile recuperative state. This is especially so during cold and flu season. A simple bad cold can turn devastating, at the very least it will make us twice as miserable as the normal person due to dry mouth conditions and being forced to breathe through your mouth. Take my word for it a simple cold, even years after cancer, if you have severely damaged salivary glands is an absolutely horrible experience. It may seem a little extreme but as noted in *Keeping a Light On* I frequently wore a surgical mask when I was out, whether in a store or even when making trips up to the hospital (Lot of sick people there). You can make up little "I'm Not Contagious I'm a Cancer Treatment Survivor" stickers to wear and that makes it all better. Trust me, you will find that instead of people swerving away because you are wearing a surgical mask, or looking at you with sympathy if you have an "I'm not contagious I have Cancer sticker" (idea copyright notation?), when people see that "I'm not contagious I survived Cancer Treatments" they meet your eyes and you see encouragement and good wishes.

IF YOU ARE OUT AND ABOUT IN PUBLIC A SURGICAL MASK AND FREQUENT HAND WASHING FOR EXTRA PROTECTION CAN BE A GOOD IDEA, ESPECIALLY IF IT IS COLD AND FLU SEASON.

Try to limit exposure to extreme temperature changes in weather, and avoid coming and going from warm to cold environments without dressing adequately and appropriately. This is another avenue for the common cold to take hold. I was forced to stay inside a lot because the weather was pretty cold and inclement since I finished in January. The cold was just brutal and would get me chilled right to my bones so much so that it hurt. I was two weeks post treatment, not even close to on the way to feeling better yet when I started asking to make the trip down to the barn to see Jake and Earnhardt's Proverbs (Earnie), my two horses. Everyone knew once I got an idea in my head you couldn't convince me otherwise. I had decided I needed to see my horses and those that know me best knew if they didn't help me it would just a matter of time before I would try sneaking out on my own. Better I go down with some help than try to sneak out in my pajamas and get pneumonia. I got my way one weekend in February when sunshine and slightly warmer temperatures came together and cooperated and we kind of made it a family affair with everyone present going down together. I had not seen them at all for even the briefest period in two months. While it would still be a long time before I was ready to haul feed or clean stalls it sure felt good to walk into the barn and breathe in the horsey hay smells, hug their strong warm necks and soak up some horse energy. I wish we had thought of videotaping the reunion because it was quite touching. They were very vocal when they saw me, especially my Jake. Their obvious happiness, the gentle nudges and low whickers of concern, warmed my heart and reminded me that even if my kids were grown, I still had my other kids waiting on me to get better.

Before you know it you will barely feel like you have had a break at all because appointments for follow ups will have you running around quite regularly again, so much so that you will probably get irritated at having so many to go to. After your initial follow up, which would normally be within that first week of finishing treatments, there may be appointments with each of the individual doctors on your team approximately every two weeks. It would be rare indeed to get all of your appointments with every doctor scheduled on the same day, so as you can see that this translates into quite a few appointments per month.

Not as rigorous as daily treatments no, but quite frankly by the time I was finally starting to really feel a little better I was getting pretty irritated with so many trips and so much time spent driving up there to hear everyone say the same thing. Chemo doctor after reviewing latest blood test results: "Looking good", ENT doctor "keep up the good work" and Dr. B. "see you in a couple of weeks". Even worse though, follow up trips for two out of the three doctors always included a look at my throat. This was done regularly during post treatment follow up with a camera at the end of a thin flexible tube that delivered video feed pictures to a computer screen. It wasn't that the scope procedure really hurt that bothered me, the examination is not really painful as long as your doctor knows what he is doing, it was more because of the numbing spray used. That stuff was just so extremely foul and nasty tasting, to the point of almost causing vomiting. Yuck hair standing on end remembering it. Not only that the terrible taste would last for hours and hours beyond the actual few minutes of the appointments and leave me with a very dry sore throat for the whole rest of the day, no matter how much water I drank.

This was the norm for me and probably for most survivors for almost six months. Follow up appointments will continue pretty close together until after the first clean PET scan or a cancer free diagnosis is given. In most cases over time follow ups will lengthen to a month between visits and then three months and eventually six months until finally you will be able to go a whole year between

check-ups. I am getting ahead of our recuperation /
recovery period though, I promised to tell the PEG Tube
story which fits in before we reach that point. Readers with
Head/neck or throat cancers, who do have a PEG tube,
will want to know the PEG tube details.

It had taken me a while but by the end of April I was
actually starting to feel a bit better strength wise, I felt like I
was rounding the bend, except for a couple of things
holding me back. First of all my neck had begun to become
increasingly quite painful. This situation had been
continuing to deteriorate for a while. Range of mobility had
been rapidly decreasing and it was difficult to turn my head
to either side, look up or down, and even keeping it
balanced precariously up there on top of my wobbly neck
seemed a challenge some days. There was no quick fix for
my neck, I would eventually begin physical therapy in the
not too distant future, but the other thing I had decided
was really holding me back was that PEG tube, and that
was something I felt could be changed pretty quickly. Just
get rid of it and that will get rid of that pain and let the hole
heal. The PEG site had become very painful, with the tube
pulling and pinching sharply with every move I made. It
was most irritating of all while I was walking, it made me
still feel like such an invalid. I had to walk real careful and
adjust my posture to a slightly hunched over position
(which contributed to neck pain) just so that the skin of my
stomach wasn't stretched taught by standing too erect. The
way I saw it the PEG tube had to go, it hurt and it was
negatively impacting posture which was in turn worse for
my neck. I was more worried about my neck and I wasn't
even using the PEG tube anymore anyway. I wanted it
gone.

I first asked my ENT in early March about removing
the PEG tube, since the doctor that put it in the year

before said it would be up to him to remove it. I had also been told before that surgery that my ENT would be able to remove it right in his office. I did worry a bit about whether it would hurt or not, it didn't seem like it would be that easy... but I figured it couldn't hurt any worse in the long run than the pain it caused on a daily basis. After researching PEG Tube removal online it sounded pretty simple. I read that it could be done in the office and that all the doctor had to do was deflate the little balloon bumper inside my belly and he would be able to pull the tube right out through the hole. The first time I asked my ENT in the beginning of March he said he could remove it in the office, but outright refused to remove it yet. He said he was still concerned I could take a turn for the worse.

At my next appointment with him in the end of March I asked again would he remove he PEG Tube? I was again told no. I made it very clear to him the PEG tube was causing me a lot of pain. Every move pulled and burned, the skin around it had become inflamed from stomach acid leakage even though I had cared for it very carefully, keeping it clean and using the provided special pink cream. I told him I was no longer even using it, and that it was making my neck worse because it affected my posture. He still said "no", that we would talk about it at the next appointment. I came in again first half of April, déjà vu, he was still insisting he would not take it out yet, that he could be sued for medical malpractice if anything happened and I needed it later. I again tried to explain very clearly just how aggravating, painful and useless the thing had become to me, but he stuck with no that day. I really got quite worked up and was pretty forceful about insisting I needed it gone. He said to remind him at my next appointment and if I was still so insistent he would take it out. Remind him? As if I was going to let him forget. I went out of that office fuming mad that day.

When I returned for the next follow up at the end of April it seemed like I waited an extra long time before being called back into the treatment area. I think he knew I was going to remind him and they were trying to have fewer patients out in the waiting room to hear me. I had already decided in my mind that I was not leaving with that PEG tube still in place torturing me and hindering my every move. All of the doctors sympathized and had acknowledged that skinny people did tend to have more problems with PEG Tube discomfort over the long term because of pulling, but none of them thought the pain outweighed the risk of removing it, just in case I needed it. When I went back he again tried to go with the same old song and dance, and still did not want to remove it yet, bringing up how he could be accused of medical malpractice if he did and I needed it later. He said he was going to make my next appointment for one month since I seemed to be doing well. I was not going home with that PEG Tube for another month! I think that is what really did it for me. A month? No way. He had said he would consider taking it out, I had already had enough pain from it and was so looking forward to it gone, he couldn't say no. To the shock of my husband and the doctor, his nurse and myself I said "I'm not leaving with this thing still in" and started opening drawers looking around for scissors, I told him "Fine I guess after I cut the end off of this someone else will have to do surgery to get the rest of it out". I guess I was pretty convincing, because it was a pretty short standoff. He asked one more time if he could convince me to "just wait till the next appointment", to which I quickly replied "no way am I walking out with this burning cigar head pressed into my side for another month". After a moment he relented, saying fine, I would have to sign an AMA against Medical Advice release waiver, he would take it out. He told me take a seat on the exam table, he would be right back, it would take a few minutes to get the Medical release paperwork ready. At this point I was thinking I won, but I was also wondering how he was going to deflate the little balloon and hoping it didn't hurt too badly pulling it out. I had a few minutes to sweat and worry a bit about it, but all in all as nervous as I was, I was still really glad I was getting it out, and said so to my husband. He was still a little mad at me for acting crazy and making a scene.

When the doctor came back in I had a hard time reading him, we had gotten along well throughout the treatments we just didn't agree over the PEG Tube. I knew I was right, I needed it gone. It was hard to tell, did he look more like I had really pissed him off? Or was he really feeling sorry for me because he knew what was coming better than I did? He asked if I knew it was going to hurt, and I said I figured as much, but still insisted it would be better to get it over with, than continue to hurt everyday for another whole month. I signed the paperwork along with the witnesses. He told me to lay flat on the table and I did. I kind of propped my head up a little with my arms and the thin hospital pillow, trying to get a better view of my stomach, thinking I am finally going to see how he deflates this balloon. He and the nurse had put on fresh gloves and were preparing sterile packing material and strips of really heavy paper backed thick rubber tape, like you would expect to see for broken ribs. They rolled the tray over to the examining table where I was laying with my belly exposed, they were ready to start. He placed one gloved hand down on my belly with the tube threaded through his fingers and pressed down very firmly, telling me it was very important to hold still. He said "ready?"... I was about to say "wait a minute isn't there a balloon you have to deflate first"? He pulled. It was like a gun had been shot from the inside of my belly outward. There are no words to describe the pain. It was so intense I saw stars and just wow, speechless, thankfully the worst of it passed pretty quickly, diminishing from a ripping gunshot wound to a throbbing hot pain within a few minutes. I think I came pretty close to passing out. The doctor continued applying strong pressure with his hand and the packing material and encouraging me to "breathe deep, keep breathing", I opened my eyes and mumbled "I thought there was going to be a balloon to deflate?" He said no he had known all along the model I had was a solid rubber bumper.

As they were tightly wrapping me in the heavy tape, that I was not to touch or remove for three days, I finally understood why he had kept putting it off. He wasn't such a bad guy he just knew that it would hurt like hell. Eventually they probably would have scheduled a one day surgery after approval by the insurance company to remove the PEG tube with some kind of general anesthesia, IF I had waited... but I really could not wait anymore. If you are tough enough and want it bad enough it can be removed without general anesthesia in the office, I'm living proof of that, but be careful what you wish for.

IF YOU HAVE A PEG TUBE ASK YOUR DOCTOR TO EXPLAIN WHAT TYPE YOU HAVE AND WHAT IT WILL IT BE LIKE WHEN IT IS REMOVED.

All in all as bad as it did hurt at the moment by the next day I was very happy it was gone and I was able to at least stand up straighter. I was glad I did it. It was after that point that I really owned being a survivor I think. That

PEG Tube was such a painful constant reminder of being a patient, and just did not fit in with being a survivor with spring weather coming.

Aside from continuing to take extra good care of your skin and oral cavity and ensuring proper rest and hydration, nutrition is as always important as well. As suggested earlier experiment with foods and find what says eat me for you. Dry mouth, damaged taste buds, and a not so hearty constitution may dictate what you actually *enjoy* eating for quite some time, but of course you must eat well. You will find after a while sugars will probably no longer taste as bad, in fact they may have almost no taste at all. This is actually a problem. At least when sugars had a bad taste we automatically avoided them, but as we reach a point where we can't really taste them, they are not as offensive, and we are more likely to consume them in our every day diet. I am not going to offer a lot of advice about eating other than to keep in mind a super high sugar diet is not best, I would rather you experiment for yourself.

I will say in the early stages of recovery for quite some time there was nothing I really liked to eat, it tasted nasty, felt nasty in my mouth, or was hard to swallow. I ate a lot of mashed potatoes with gravy and vegetables. I say experiment though because that is how I came across the first post treatment dish that actually made me say I recognize that and I like it. I fried up some thick sliced portabella mushrooms with garlic cloves in butter and added a little sprinkle of squeezed lemon juice over the top after they were done. My goodness you would think I had just discovered the most delicious of cakes and pastries or the juiciest, most tender New York strip the way I was Ummmming over that dish that day. It is such a surprise and a treat when you find something new you put in your mouth that makes you go oooh that's good. As noted it is unfortunately true that dry mouth and damage to the taste bud sensors can be long term.

CHALLENGE YOUR TASTE BUDS, TRY TO WAKE THEM UP, STIMULATE THEM AND YOUR SALIVARY GLANDS BY INTRODUCING A VARIETY OF FLAVORS, ESPECIALLY SOURS AND BITTERS.

Damage to salivary glands and the return of properly functioning taste bud sensors on the tongue probably rate pretty low on the list of things that are being worried about early on in the recuperative period; but in the long run this issue can actually be among the longest lasting and one of the most detrimental quality of life concern faced by cancer survivors. It may not rank as the most troublesome issue encountered by head/neck throat cancer survivors, but it is probably the most common. Salivary gland function is also one of the main reasons the two year mark is considered so important to take notice of. I experienced a continued decrease in salivary gland production for months and months post treatment. By the time I was a year beyond treatment I had reached a point of extreme dry mouth, to the point it affected my ability to be outside for extended periods of time. This was especially true in hot weather. This remained unimproved for some time. It was at the two year mark that my radiation doctor shocked me a bit.

We were discussing just how poorly my salivary glands had recovered, the problems I associated with the issue and the various topical sprays and mouthwashes available. I found that none of these had really provided the true moisture I really needed and they failed to achieve relief of the radiation induced dry mouth symptoms adequately enough to be the active outdoor lifestyle person I wanted to return to being. I mentioned I was looking forward to when function improved and that was when he let me know that he really did not expect there to be any further improvement. In other words he did not feel I could look forward to production of any additional saliva. The almost nonexistent, rather thick consistency moisture I was able to very scantily produce was about the best I could expect, and he warned it could become even less over time. There was so little I couldn't imagine it could get any less.

THE TWO YEAR MARK IS CONSIDERED BY MANY PHYSICIANS TO BE THE POINT OF OPTIMUM POST TREATMENT RECOVERY, ESPECIALLY IN REGARDS TO RETURN OF FUNCTION OF THE SALIVARY GLANDS.

The dry mouth was bad, but had been manageable within reason by introducing liquids. I had already been carrying a water bottle absolutely everywhere I went. I mean really and literally everywhere. I learned quickly failure to keep that water bottle with me at all times when outside would result in chapped dry cracked lips and sores from the insides of my lips and mouth sticking to my teeth. What really bothered me the most though as I was trying to move on through recovery and beyond was not just the dry mouth environment, but the dry throat and airways I suffered from. Upon exertion which brought about an increase in adrenaline, in short doing anything that was fun or hard work, I found that my throat and airways became as dried out as my mouth almost immediately. Inhaling became difficult and it would burn as I breathed in and the air rushed passed through my dry airways. I would have to, and still do, stop what I am doing and retreat inside and resort to sitting in front of a steam vaporizer with a towel over my head trying to re moisturize my throat. Since it was worse in summer and I was usually so hot I bought a cool air mist vaporizers too. This quality of life concern seemed to be completely overlooked, ignored or perhaps it is under reported by survivors? I tried to discuss with one of my doctors an idea I had to help relieve the "problem", but he did not seem to even understand the "problem", like others he recommended the available dry mouth washes, rinses and sprays. No one else but me and other survivors who have felt well enough to try to return to engaging in outdoor activities and competitive fun seem to even know this quality of life issue exist. It is very distressing when trying to breath and each inhalation is like pulling burning hot daggers down your throat. Worse than that, the sides of your throat can get so dry they stick together upon swallowing. I have had a number of quite scary choking episodes. For me this has been the greatest negative impact as far as I am concerned in regards to quality of life. I have been unable to enjoy a real return to working with and riding my horses, mainly because it takes some time and effort to groom and saddle up for a ride and I find that by the time the half hour or so has passed that it takes me to accomplish the preparation my mouth and throat are absolutely beyond parched. You can drink water to wet your mouth, but you cannot inhale liquid to soothe dry tortured airways.

DRY MOUTH AND THE LESSER KNOWN DRY AIRWAYS CONDITION CAN AFFECT QUALITY OF LIFE AND IF PRESENT AT THE TWO YEAR RECOVERY MARK UNFORUNATELY MAY BE A PERMANENT LIFETIME CONDITION.

I had also mentioned at about four months post treatment I had been having quite a bit of trouble with pain in my neck, this continued and by the fifth month the pain extended down into my back, with range of motion becoming progressively more restricted. At six months post treatment on a beautiful summer day in July I went for my first PET scan and received the good news later that same day, it was clean. My lab results for blood tests had been well within acceptable ranges as well. For the first time in almost a year my doctors told me I was cancer free. I had become a cancer survivor, officially. I entered physical therapy and rehabilitation for my neck shortly after that.

It took quite some time, but with regular appointments utilizing therapies such as passive stretching, electrical stimulation and applied traction, as well as performing the recommended exercises at home I did see major improvement with a decrease in pain as long as I did not over tax myself and range of motion was much better by the end of the first year.

DO NOT BE DISHEARTENED IF YOU FIND YOU HAVE TO GO TO PHYSICAL REHABILITATIVE THERAPY, MANY POST TREATMENT SURVIVORS NEED TO. IT IS HARD WORK BUT IT WILL PAY OFF.

I have a few favorite ways to exercise and try to keep things loose. One is by listening to music. I have always loved all kinds of music; it is like universal medicine for the body and soul. Those rusty dance moves are great for your body. Just dance like no one is watching, and hopefully they aren't, it's good for you no matter how old or how young you are. Singing is great for vocal chords, (if my usually loud happy monotone could be considered that) and very good exercise for the muscles of the throat and larynx. You may not sound any better than the dance moves looked, but it's good for you. Lastly for my neck I most enjoy standing on the deck off the back of the house and gazing up at a star filled sky late at night. I also noticed as I moved further beyond treatments that my balance did not seem as good, so I started to throw in some different yoga position balance moves as well. I kind of like to challenge and at times embarrass myself from home using my rudimentary knowledge and my own sense of knowing my body but others may find it preferable to join a more directed or focused exercise or yoga group. All is good, the important thing is that we want to keep trying to slowly rebuild our bodies gently. Radiation treatments, especially of the head/neck and throat can cause severe and lasting damage, and unfortunately even years after treatments end can problems can surface. You will need a lifetime of monitoring as far as the radiation treatment aspect of life beyond cancer, and this will be discussed further in the next chapter.

Besides the after effects of the radiation treatments upon muscle, tissues and bone there may also be nerve damage that is usually specifically associated with chemotherapy treatments. Nerve damage can cause tingling, or numbness in the extremities. I experienced some numbness in my hands, which resolved within the first few months after chemotherapy treatments ended on its own. I also experienced electrical shock like sensations that traveled from my neck to my toes. It would happen when I looked downward if I was sitting or standing in a fairly nice straight posture. It was almost the same type of feeling like when you put your tongue on a nine volt battery, except that it would go from the back the head all the way down the spine and into the legs, right to the feet. I had at first thought it was all part of the problem with my neck and due to the radiation treatments but both of those doctors said no that it was a symptom of nerve damage from the chemotherapy. It was a strange sensation to say the least. I would not exactly say painful, but literally it was a shocking sensation. It did last for quite a while, eventually by the end of the first year it had almost stopped, and was only occasionally happening every so often. By the end of the second year I had stopped experiencing the electrical shock sensations except for very rare occasions.

Another problem commonly related to chemotherapy is tinnitus, or ringing in the ears. Oh my goodness I wish I could tell you that has gotten better over time. I have in general tried to stay upbeat and I am sure you are aware I have kind of glossed over the pain and misery parts of early recovery, but I have stayed truthful. I must say if I told you the ringing in my ears was any better two years later I would be a liar. My ears to this day ring so bad I have trouble hearing clearly, especially when there is more than one sound. For example when there is a group of people and there is more than one person talking at once or when a movie has loud sound effects or musical accompaniment I have trouble hearing the words. I have learned to live with it, preferring not to risk making it worse. I know of people who have tried medications and even surgery to correct this but at this time I do not personally know of a single person who was suffering from tinnitus who has successfully overcome the problem with either method. Much like salivary gland function this too seems to be one of the after effects that if present at the two year mark will most likely continue or possibly worsen over the long term. Speaking of ears, I have literarily talked yours off and it is time to be moving along, beyond the two year maximum recovery point, time to jump ahead into the future and years of *Living Life Beyond Cancer.* Hopefully the advice offered thus far will offer some degree of assistance and guidance to others as they journey through treatment and recovery.

I have tried to encompass and convey the overall cancer experience; I speak with the voice of a stage IVB Throat cancer survivor, therefore I regret there may be challenges and obstacles I was less familiar with and left uncovered, but I also hope though that there are many more who will find that some of the advice and information was not needed at all.

11 LIFE BEYOND CANCER

Is there Life after Cancer, can we really be happy or satisfied as cancer survivors? These are very personal questions that each of us will have to confront in our own time and our own way, bridges that we will cross when they are reached, we may balk and buck but sooner or later we must push forward and cross those bridges as we come upon them and choose the path that embraces life.

THE ANSWER TO WHETHER ONE CAN TRULY BE HAPPY OR SATISFIED LIVING LIFE AS A CANCER SURVIVOR CAN BE AS SIMPLE AND AS COMPLICATED AS ASKING ONE QUESTION, "WERE WE HAPPY OR SATISFIED WITH OUR LIVES BEFORE WE WERE DIAGNOSED"?

Our health is very important as we continue through the years beyond that two year recovery point. It is possible we may experience lifetime post cancer related issues, we may also have, or develop in the future, health problems that are completely separate from or co existing with the post cancer effects. You may be fortunate enough that you feel great and see doctors at a bare minimum per year, or unfortunately you may feel like you are being put back onto the merry go round ride discussed in Life Before Cancer.

YOU ARE A CANCER SURVIVOR, CANCER FREE, REMEMBER AND USE THE ADVICE AND TIPS FOUND IN *LIFE BEFORE CANCER*, STAY IN TOUCH WITH YOUR BODY AND STAY PRO ACTIVE IN YOUR HEALTH CARE.

Specific health concerns encountered by individuals post cancer treatments, given the diversity of cancer types and locations and treatment options available, including taking into account the individuality of each person, as previously discussed in chapter 4 *State of Mind* would be an immense topic that I am not sure an entire book devoted to could encompass or do justice. There are so many types and locations and treatments of and for cancer that the overall outcomes of each person are always very individual. While some of the more common health concerns will be discussed it will mainly be in reference to the limitations they may impose upon us overall as we move forward into Life Beyond Cancer.

The thing is where do we move forward to? We can begin by asking; "Were we happy where we were before the cancer diagnosis?" If this question gets an immediate no, without requiring a lot of thought, then perhaps now will be the time to find out what really will make you happy? If everything happens for a reason then maybe there is something else we should be trying to do or getting involved in?

If we were happy before cancer the next question is "Can we go back to doing it"? Before cancer were we working? Was it strenuous? Were we in an inside or an outside environment? Did we have professional careers and if so were they highly stressful and did they involve long hours? Were we in school or retired? Will limitations post cancer make it difficult or impossible to return to doing whatever it was that was done prior to being diagnosed? Can we return to doing everything we used to do that we were happy with? Not just from a work or career aspect but from a pleasure and leisure time perspective as well. It is very possible the answer may be no, to one degree or another. Even individuals who did have jobs that were less strenuous and performed inside in a climate controlled environment may experience great difficulties when trying to return to work because much of this work involves sitting or standing for long periods of time.

RECURRING NECK AND BACK PROBLEMS CAN PLAGUE SOME HEAD/NECK AND THROAT CANCER SURVIVORS FOR LIFE

I did think I enjoyed what I was doing and would have gladly returned to what I was used to, but over the past few years I have had to return for additional physical rehabilitation therapy twice, both times so far have thankfully eventually produced improvements and positive results. I also had to have surgery to repair a torn ligament between my neck and shoulder at one point. Aside from neck and back problems I fatigue very easily, am prone to headaches, I am unable to produce saliva and I have frequent stomach issues, so can I return to being a construction painting contractor and work outside and haul ladders and five gallon buckets of paint like I used to do? No, absolutely not. Ups and downs and bridges to cross you know.

HAPPINESS AND SATISFACTION CANNOT BE BASED SOLELY ON THE ABILITY TO RETURN TO DOING EVERYTHING WE DID BEFORE CANCER REMEMBER TO BE GRATEFUL FOR WHAT WE CAN STILL DO.

State of Mind, how happy you are, how satisfied you are, can play a key role in how healthy you actually are and feel. When you wake up in the morning are you happy to see sunshine peeking through the blinds or are you rolling over and pulling the blankets over your head? Sometimes achieving happiness and satisfaction is not about overcoming the physical challenges we face that keep us from doing what we used to do, or want to do or feel that we need to do, some limitations are permanent and cannot be overcome no matter how hard we try, and if doing everything we did before was the only way to be happy or satisfied we could be set up to fail. Instead we must be able to make and accept changes in our lifestyle that adapt to our limitations.

ENERGY LEVELS, MUSCLE MASS, OVERALL STRENGTH AND STAMINA MAY NEVER BOUNCE BACK COMPLETELY TO PRE CANCER CAPABILITIES.

This is another one of those important points that I think is somewhat overlooked and/or underrated by many, except the cancer survivors themselves, who tend to figure it out on their own. Quite often, depending on how advanced the cancer was, how aggressive the treatments were, the strengths and dosages used for the chemotherapy and or radiation treatments, we are not and never will be the same physical person we used to be.

Yes I said it, I am able to admit, accept and live with that now. There was a time that this was not so though, I used to push and push and wear myself out. I know that dropping and banging out 25-50 push-ups in proper form without breaking a sweat like I could seven-eight years ago is only a memory. I also know that a year or two ago I would have pushed myself to do ten if I was challenged to do so, I would still maintain proper form, but it would be with great effort. Now I am smart enough to settle for five when I exercise. All throughout my third year post treatments I pushed myself hard, hey when you're exercising the motto is no pain no gain right? Well, there has been plenty of pain, but I have not been able to regain my muscle mass, and my weight continues to hover a hair above the one hundred pound mark on the scale no matter how hard I try to gain.

YOU CAN PUSH TOO HARD AND WANT TOO MUCH.

What I personally experienced, and have discussed with other cancer survivors is that beyond the two year peak mark many of us did see some continued further improvements, such as strength and stamina, and foods tasting better that continued into the third year if we worked for it, but beyond that point it seemed to feel like we had reached a plateau, and pushing hard and over exerting tended to wear down instead of building up.

IT WILL TAKE TIME BUT LEARN YOUR LIMITS AND REMEMBER NOT TO PUSH YOUR BODY BEYOND THEM

I have spoken with a number of people who feel, as I began to, that the fourth year seemed like the beginning of a very slow gradual decline in strength and stamina if we pushed too much. It wasn't so much that I (we) grew weaker, it was more like we tried to do more as time passed, or maybe more was expected of us by those around us, and we would try to do these things. Problem is we would over extend and wear ourselves out to the point we were so sore and so tired it would take days of recuperation afterwards and sometimes worse we could pull or injure something that would take even longer to stop hurting. Slow and steady wins the race. I find that I can do things, I go down to the barn every day and I feed the chickens and rabbits and the goat and the horses and I can even clean stalls, but I have to do it at my pace and I have to use my body muscles carefully wisely, building and maintaining, instead of over working or incorrectly stretching. My neck continues to be troublesome even all these years later and requires that I am always careful just how quickly I move and in which direction. I have learned the hard way over the years that a wrong, too quick move can cause severe pain and require a lengthy rest/recovery period, and even physical therapy. This is why I say in these years beyond cancer try to stay within certain pain limits, but at the same time move and use things to retain the mobility and range of motion that we do have.

THIS IS ONE OF THOSE INDIVIDUAL ASPECTS OF CANCER THAT EACH WILL HAVE TO FEEL THEIR OWN WAY THROUGH; LISTEN TO YOUR BODY, IT WILL TELL YOU WHETHER IT IS OKAY WITH WHAT YOU ARE TRYING TO DO.

I would also like to say do not let my own personal experiences discourage you from striving to build back up to pre cancer status, every case, every person is individual. As I have said I do know people who bounce back. Half of my problem is that I am attempting to return to a very demanding outdoor, heavy lifting, pre cancer status, not everyone is trying to do the same. You might not have been able to load hay bales or sling 50 pound sacks of grain into the back of a pickup truck before cancer, so of course you wouldn't be working towards being able to do that post cancer (although you could make it your goal if you chose to I guess). Pain will most likely be a problem I will always have to cope with due to the target area of the radiation treatments.

Another reason I think others may have different or perhaps more satisfactory results returning to post cancer status is because in my case I have a combination of factors that go right along with trying to return to doing such hard physical work. I am middle aged; older people do not regenerate cells as quickly as the very young. I underwent a very aggressive maximum dosage double whammy treatment course against a very late stage cancer. My thyroid does not properly function and continues to create some issues. Also, before I was diagnosed with cancer, I underwent a total hysterectomy. So I would say it is very possible age, lowered or imbalanced hormone levels, on top of such an aggressive treatment course could be contributing factors.

Aside from limitations imposed by the dry mouth and dry throat conditions there are other Post Radiation treatment problems that may surface years later. Some of which may cause moderate to severe pain, and others that are very serious.

IT IS VERY IMPORTANT THAT YOU CONTINUE TO BE MONITORED FOR POST RADIATION TREATMENT EFFECTS FOR THE REST OF YOUR LIFE.

This goes for everyone who underwent radiation treatments but for Head/Neck and throat cancer survivors this is especially important because the target area of treatment generally involved the brain and neck, both of which are very important. I am not going to go into additional detail here about the really scary stuff… these are bridges we will cross if we come to them, the important thing is to continue to monitor closely. Post radiation treatment effects and symptoms aside from dry mouth vary greatly and may include anything from joint pain to balance issues, vision problems and/or memory loss, etc… This can be due to areas of muscle atrophy and possible necrosis (dead tissue) within the old target zones, especially the neck, jaw and throat muscles which are prone to becoming troublesome many years later. Sometimes these problems may be related to circulatory issues or the necrotic tissue from within the old target area. I do not want to be a Debbie Downer, but after maximum dosage radiation treatments for a head/neck throat cancer I must confess my neck and back continue to be a very painful reminder that will require close monitoring as time passes.

Dental health and decay problems are another common concern that can develop years and years after the end of the treatments.

YOU WILL NEED TO MAINTAIN A VERY CLOSE RELATIONSHIP WITH YOUR DENTIST.

If you find you are running into a lot of problems with dental health, (There is no pain more excruciating that tooth aches) you are not alone, this is common for those without natural saliva. You may have to make drastic decisions down the road, yet another of those bridges you may come upon. This could even include considering dentures, as I have done. If a dentist talks to you about implant teeth knowing that you have had head/neck or throat cancer radiation treatments I personally would recommend that you find another dentist that is highly experienced in post radiation dentistry before proceeding. At the very least get a second opinion. We have years and years ahead of us, a conservative less intrusive approach into already weakened bones, such as of the jaw line is best, in my humble opinion.

If as time passes you do feel that you are in some ways physically declining moving through these years beyond cancer it is not necessarily one of the more worrisome after effects of radiation treatments making themselves known, but may be another more manageable issue. It is quite possible if one does experience a noticeable slowing down at some point beyond the two or more year mark it may simply be an indication of a chemical imbalance or deficiency, many of which can be alleviated or corrected through medication, diet, or perhaps some physical therapy is in order. It could even be that you are having other medical issues not directly cancer related. Keep in touch with your body, get a good primary care physician you trust and keep on requesting copies of those blood test results.

Over the years as a cancer survivor I have encountered a number of situations that required medical attention. Of course as a cancer survivor, even after years pass, when we do not feel good we can't help it, we start thinking "is it back?" During the first two to three years post treatment every concern I had was laid down at the feet of my oncology team, but after a few years, as we move further along we are only seeing them on average once per year. That is why it is important that we have a primary care physician that we trust and that understands our concerns as we move beyond those close ties with our oncologists. Pop up medical issues can really cause major worry and survivors need to get to the bottom of what is going on and get our answers ASAP so we can stop worrying.

IF YOU WERE NOT SATISFIED WITH YOUR PRIMARY CARE PHYSICIAN PRIOR TO DIAGNOSIS YOU NEED TO FIND ONE YOU WORK WELL WITH WHO UNDERSTANDS YOU. MOVING BEYOND THE 3-4 YEAR MARK AS CANCER SURVIVOR THIS IS MORE IMPORTANT THAN EVER.

Over the years post treatment I have been diagnosed with kidney stones, which have flared up and resolved/passed twice now. Apparently due to the chemotherapy I received my kidneys do not function at optimum capacity, I am not sure but others may encounter this issue as well. My kidneys are not so bad that they are a cause of major concern. I am not to use NSAID's or Ibuprofen medicines at all, and I remain prone to developing stones occasionally now and then. While the experience was painful, both times the stones did manage to pass. The biggest scare was that during the first episode while one of the tests to check my kidneys was being done there were lesions noted on my urinary bladder. This was cause for concern and I did have to go in for a biopsy. Just hearing the word biopsy OMG, yes, that was no fun. My primary care doctor had the one day surgery arranged within a week, knowing that I was of course worried. I am happy to say that those tests came back as benign and the urologist said the lesions were of no concern. About a year after that I also had to have my gall bladder removed. After enduring a few months of misery, during which I had halfway convinced myself "it must be back", I finally consented to undergoing the many tests my primary ordered. I am always leery of getting stuck back on that merry go round and I did get quite irritated that it took three separate tests over the course of a two month period to figure out the problem, but it was finally determined my gall bladder was inflamed, not working properly, and needed to go. I must confess I did feel better after I recovered from that, but to this day digestion issues continue to play random havoc, and I do occasionally have some days that are so bad I am temporarily incapacitated. Lacking saliva may be a contributing factor to some digestive problems because there are enzymes in our saliva that help to break down food. Also food itself is more difficult to eat without saliva. Small bites and chew well as Mom used to say is good advice. I also had to have my shoulder repaired as mentioned earlier, but at least that bump in the road didn't scare me.

REGULAR BLOOD WORK SHOULD CONTINUE AND BE DONE MINIMUM EVERY SIX MONTHS TO MONITOR MAJOR BODILY FUNCTIONS.

Regularly scheduled blood tests are generally under the direction of your chemotherapy doctor or your primary care physician. Radiation treatments require lifetime follow up, but my chemotherapy oncologist told me he expected me to come to him for lab testing for a full five years. Blood tests are done to continue to monitor levels of important bodily functions and can be a barometer of health. For example lab work can check the performance of kidneys and liver, and very important in the case of head/neck and throat cancer survivors the function of the thyroid gland. This one little gland can play chaos with your life, affecting appetite and causing weight gain or weight loss, sleep disorders and fatigue, and the list goes on and on. Often the thyroid gland is totally destroyed by the radiation treatments, but luckily this can be corrected with careful monitoring and use of a medication known generically as levothyroxine. My thyroid has sputtered back and forth into fits of production and decline over the years, as it continues to try to produce the hormones and create the chemical conversions it is supposed to. When this does happen I feel the effects. You know those ups and downs we were talking about? Well the thyroid can be one of the biggest causes of these. The thyroid can be tricky with many symptoms that could be something else, ranging from inability to sleep to being too sleepy to suffering severe muscle cramps especially in my legs, to a lack of appetite and energy, and many others. Now that I have come to recognize symptoms sooner I can somewhat shorten the down periods. Usually a simple blood test will determine if an adjustment is needed, and the doctor will counter with a decrease or increase in the medication as needed. Sometimes it can still take months to get back into normal ranges. This is just one of many reasons to continue to be pro active and keep up with those lab appointments.

MANY CHEMOTHERAPY ONCOLOGIST D OCTORS WILL TELL YOU THAT THEY EXPECT TO SEE YOU FOR A FULL 5 YEARS.

Dry mouth and dry airways can severely hamper activities and exertion, especially those taking place in an outdoor environment. By the end of my third year I never did see any further improvement in salivary production, I guess the doctor was right about that two year peak recovery mark. In fact the dry mouth dry airways problem has not only persisted, but as many may find, it can actually become even worse post two year mark. To this very day dry mouth and dry airways continues to be the most consistent devastating, life altering and limiting of the post cancer treatment effects I cope with. Bodily pain I find varies in level from day to day with some days better than others, but the dry mouth is the same dry mouth every day. It may seem a small price to pay compared to the possible outcomes; death, losing the ability to speak, or to swallow, and I do remember to be grateful, but between pain and the dry mouth and airways I am very severely limited in my ability to comfortably remain outside and engage in demanding or energetic activities. As a lifelong outdoors person this is a very serious issue that greatly affects and negatively impacts my lifestyle and therefore my happiness.

DAMAGE TO THE SALIVARY GLANDS RESULTING IN DRY MOUTH AND THE LESSER KNOWN DRY AIRWAYS IS PROBABLY THE MOST COMMON CONCERN SHARED BETWEEN CANCER SURVIVORS, ESPECIALLY HEAD/NECK OR THROAT CANCERS.

Whether your joy was hiking, biking, jogging or playing ball or horseback riding, or riding on a motorcycle, or all the above, dry mouth and dry airways will probably bring you to a stop during these outdoors activities before you run out of available energy. Dry mouth and dry airways has

pretty much been life shattering for me. My work and my
joys, especially my horses, were all out of doors activities. I
do still try to plant a small vegetable garden each year but I
have trouble keeping up, and by mid season when it gets
really hot I have to abandon it for the most part. I usually
manage to get some early harvest of tomatoes and
cucumbers and peppers and such. My herbs thank
goodness are strong and tend to fend for themselves quite
well with the minimal care, continuing to spread year after
year. My horses are fat and happy and my hardworking still
somewhat patient husband likes to say "Must be nice to be
on a permanent vacation". Sometimes I wonder if the man
means me or the horses, we both costs him a small fortune
to keep. I know it is very hard for him to understand why
they are so very important to me, but it is enough that for
as long as we can continue he supports my wishes. Call me
weird, stubborn, selfish or all the above, I know Horse
People will get me, but I feel like there is so little of "me"
left, the "old" me, and Jake and Earnie I must keep. They
are not only a source of energy for me, they give me
purpose, keep me motivated, inspired and moving, and give
me a goal to keep working towards. Everybody needs
someone that needs them, or challenges them; I need my
horses as much as they need me. Jake and Earnie are 14
and 10 years old now, and it would truly break my heart, I
could never part with them, especially not in the all too
common animal abuse/cruelty/slaughter environment of
today. Horses have been approved for sale as dog food
now in the United States. Jake has been here since he was a
baby, and he is Earnie's daddy, she was born here delivered
right into my hands in the huge barn that my husband and
I built together when I was strong. The two horses that I
did agree to place years earlier, right after the nest emptied
and I was forced to admit that four horses for a two person

household were too many to afford (I am not unreasonable), took forever to place safely, and we continue to check on them to this day. Earnie's Mom, Brandy, was a mustang rescue from a herd out of Wyoming that I trained, and she is much loved and now almost 20 years old here in Georgia. Radar is a very athletically inclined hunter learner mount at a very upscale equestrian farm in Connecticut. I was lucky I managed to place them in great forever homes, but it was not easy and things were different back then. I keep telling Kevin that someday I will make it up to him for all the trouble Jake and Earnie and I have been, somehow I will find a way to contribute income as a productive citizen, someday he will get a chance to take a vacation. I just need to keep up the faith that everything happens for a reason, no matter how long it takes for things to turn around. I have now bored you enough with horse stuff while making it clear that permanent dry mouth from salivary gland damage is much more than an inconvenience, it can be life altering depending on your lifestyle. The horses have provided a very nice segue though to another problem besides physical challenges of Life *Beyond Cancer* that I am sure is faced by many other cancer survivors and not unique to my situation, and that is trying to stay positive and not let ourselves be dragged down by financial stress.

For me and perhaps other survivors this stress is compounded by our own frustrated feelings of ineptitude and incompetence and even guilt because we are not contributing financially or physically as we used to. These feelings are even worse when we have expensive passions that we do not want to give up, even when we cannot afford them, or even get to enjoy using them much, like owning horses. I'm the one that got sick, I'm the puny weakling that can't return to my old work and I'm the one that does not want to give up my horses. I feel like it was all my fault that we have had to use our savings.

We were always a hard working middleclass blue collar two income family before I became sick. We didn't take vacations or anything fancy but the kids had everything they needed, we made many improvements around the property over the years and the bills and the mortgages were paid on time without worries. It has not been easy keeping everything together though as more and more years post treatment pass and I have remained unproductive. Kevin works very hard as a highly qualified mechanical Maintenance Technician but there is always more cash flow outgoing than incoming. As mentioned earlier in *Staging Your Plan of Action* we did access 401 k funds when I was first diagnosed. This was to alleviate stress throughout the lengthy treatment course, at that point we did not even know if I would live. We didn't claim hardship because it would have been very complicated and delayed the process, basically it probably would have required a lawyer to accomplish that way, so we took the tax hit that went with the distribution. I did live though, and I am still living and as the years continue to pass, as careful as we have tried to be, the problem we were trying to avoid, while it was postponed quite a while, has returned with a vengeance; Financial stress. The difference is I am no longer the cancer patient who is told don't worry we'll get by. Now the savings are depleted, now I am a cancer survivor, and now I am feeling the pressure from a few quarters to produce income.

The more time that passes since treatments are finished the more people around the survivors can kind of take it for granted that we are all better, that we don't get so tired anymore and that just isn't always the case. Often I think, or at least I hope, it is just that sometimes the people who say things do not realize how much they hurt feelings when they comment to the effect that you have energy for some things … but not work. They fail to appreciate just how much effort it really does take for us to do some of the things we are doing. Usually this happens because we are trying so hard to act positive, put on a brave face and push ourselves to prove that we can do things. Maybe we have fooled them? If I could give one piece of advice to those in the peripheral life of a cancer survivor I guess I would say;

JUST BECAUSE WE SURVIVORS ENGAGE IN A BRIEF ACTIVITY, A MOMENT OF FUN OR ACCOMPLISH SOMETHING DIFFICULT OR STRENUOUS WITH A SMILE ON OUR FACES AND GOOD WILL AND CHEER IN OUR HEARTS DOES NOT MEAN THAT IT WAS PHYSICALLY EASY FOR US TO DO.

I don't think anyone, except other survivors whether cancer treatment or traumatic injury from an accident or disaster can really understand how hard it is trying to reestablish self-worth and value again as a person when you return from the brink of death as a shell, as half the person you formerly were. Again I say for some people this adjustment might not be as difficult, cancer may have been caught early, treatment not as aggressive or you may not be trying to reenter such an active physically demanding lifestyle as the one I led prior to diagnosis. For former "tough guys" like I was, being weak, being unable to do things takes a long, long time to adjust and admit to. It took me a long time but I do now admit/know I will never be able to return to doing what used to be my career, my job, as a matter of fact I find I am very limited in what I

185

can do at all. I still believe I have abilities though that will allow me to be a productive citizen, a working member of society. I believe because I have to believe, because nothing less than being productive will make me happy.

Remember I told you I was stubborn? Well I have refused to attempt to get any kind of disability payments. This has caused friction from some quarters. I feel these programs are for people who no longer have the ability to earn an income, and I feel I can be productive. There are all kinds of requirements and restrictions upon activities in order to receive the compensation. Many people will be eligible and very much do deserve to receive disability payments after surviving cancer treatments. Sometimes retirement or severance pay is available as well. I don't want those limitations imposed upon me, I want to be allowed to live my life, I want to be free to push and challenge myself as I see fit, for as long as I am able to. I do not want to be forced to not do things simply because of being worried one activity or another may cut disability eligibility. Not to mention having been self employed, while I did pay my taxes every year for social security I paid in only the minimums, and when we did inquire if I recall correctly my monthly benefit was somewhere around $296.00 per month (based on what was paid in). My mistake, my fault again, I did not pay in enough. I never really pictured anything happening to me and actually finding myself needing it so young. To me that amount would not be worth setting limits on myself, and like I said for me to be happy with life after cancer, I need to be productive. I feel the pressure from those around me who feel I should have applied for disability years ago if I can't work, or that I should have found a job by now if I think I can. They do not understand I am looking for more than a job; I am looking to get my life back. As long as my mind remains clear I do have abilities.

You may find yourself in a situation as a cancer survivor with years under your belt, needing to either bring in income or decrease outgoing cash flow, and feeling the pressure to deliver as patience around you wears as thin as the purse strings too. I know my husband is advised often to get rid of obvious luxuries that are considered less important. Of course that would be my horses because they are so expensive. The importance of keeping them is only crystal clear to me, and probably other horse people. I do try to understand that things are said because they care and worry we will not be able to pay the mortgages. I try not to let words hurt my feelings by taking them too much to heart, I know they are well meant, but it is difficult because it makes me sad too. I am trying to remain upbeat and believe everything happens for a reason, that even if I have not succeeded yet, I will and everything will be okay. I am trying to act strong, and while I certainly do not want pity, I would really appreciate a better understanding. After struggling so hard to adapt to and either over come or accept my physical limitations as a barrier to happiness, is it all for nothing unless I can manage to prove that I can earn an income?

EXPLORE INCOME PRODUCING POSSIBILITIES WITH EMPHASIS UPON WORK FROM HOME THAT UTILIZE YOUR TALENTS OR PASSIONS, CONSIDER ATTENDING COLLEGE, LET YOURSELF DREAM, EVEN WHEN OTHERS KEEP WAKING YOU UP.

I have long had a dream to become a published and popular author, but while I was healthy life kept me too busy with other things like earning a living to really get serious. I have always loved writing and long ago, in my pre cancer years I did take classes at the Redding Institute of Children's Literature. I also have attempted a couple of manuscript submissions in those early years. Without an agent it was not so easy to become a published author and actually earn money back in the day. Years ago unsolicited manuscript submissions were not a simple email, but required a number of formal steps to even be considered for a review, before being returned along with a politely worded rejected letter. I have not been idle these past few years, I made good use of a lot of my recovery time working on a few very promising outlines and progressing quite far into developing a couple, including this one, as well as a book of poetry with a political slant. I have never really managed to follow through though and completely finish one. I would write in creative fits and then get sidetracked. Sometimes by volunteer work I was participating in, and sometimes by other ideas and projects that I thought could produce income sooner. In the case of this particular book I had no choice but to keep coming back, it could not be finished until I had actually lived and experienced enough of life beyond cancer to share, that took a few extra years.

I attempted to develop an herbal tea business since I do grow many herbs here. It was a lot of hard work harvesting and drying and creating my Mother Nature To You Herbal Green Tea blends and the web site, and labels, etc. There were many details to be ironed out, but it seemed like it could actually have been a lucrative idea. I was trying to become certified organic, since I never use chemicals here, but it turned out it is quite expensive to get legal permission to use the word "organic". Around this same time Congress was working on parts of the farm bill about to be passed that caught my attention. This was while I was in the midst of building up a happy client base of repeat customers for loose leaf herbal tea. The wording of the bill set restrictions on sales beyond a 275 mile radius from my home. I was selling online with orders as far away as Puerto Rico, so a 275 mile radius would have basically killed the business. It had been exhausting, I put a lot of work into the attempt with too much outside time, very little emotional rewards, and then the concern about legality was added and in frustration I gave up on that venture. Everyone kept telling me disregard the concerns about the new law, but I was exhausted from trying by that point. It turned out that eventually when the bill finally did pass with amendments if I earned under a certain amount I would have been exempt from the additional fees to sell beyond the set radius. Harvesting large quantities of herbs, even though I was able to break up my time outside into short blocks really had been harder than I wanted to admit though and I just didn't have it in me to try again after the disappointment of almost creating a business.

During the time I was attempting to begin the herbal tea business I was also dealing with major problems with my mouth and throat from trying to be outside so much. I developed sores from my lips sticking to my teeth; I kept going hoarse, sometimes completely losing my voice from dryness, and in general was encountering a lot of throat pain and swallowing difficulties because I could not keep it moist. I had a vaporizer but in the summer heat I would come in all sweating and sit in the hot steam and almost pass out, so I bought a cold air mist vaporizer. I would constantly have to keep coming inside to sit in front of one or the other with a towel over my head for at least a half an hour at a time, just to get my throat back to the point of bearable. As I said to be honest, even if there had not been technical problems with the herbal tea business I would not have been able to continue. I was as usual stubborn though and did try to keep at the herbal tea business for a year.

EVERYTHING HAPPENS FOR A REASON

There is an old saying that necessity is the mother of invention. It was while starting the Herbal Green Tea venture, trying to be outside so much, that I conceived the idea for a device that would allow people who suffer from severe dry mouth and dry airways to alleviate/relieve parched orifices in a more thorough and convenient hands free manner. First I had to learn about the patent process and then I had to find my way around the patent office, and then I made my way through the steps and eventually obtained a provisional patent. Before that year expired we then hired a law firm and spent money we could ill afford in the lengthy process to further develop the idea and obtained the non provisional patent protection which is now in force for the device that I call OASSISS© Oral Assistance System Supplementing Inhibited Salivary Secretion©. For the longest time I have been instructed to be secretive, and of course sign non disclosures if I spoke with anyone, but desperate times call for desperate measures, so I am openly discussing the concept but must leave out the details. So far as with everything else I have tried to do, I have cost more money and failed to produce income yet.

I do remain positive and patient with this process though because I know it takes time and that there is great value in the patent. I have absolute faith this is a great and new and unique product and any patent vultures will be in for a solid fight. The attorney continues to remind us to watch for any similar product entering the market (he thinks the patent/idea has a lot of merit and he knew what he was doing when he wrote up the claims). If so I am to let him know because then there would be an infringement suit brought.

Talk about frustrating? This simple device could potentially solve my dilemma over being productive and producing income, I could be happy. Even more importantly it would allow me, and others suffering radiation induced permanent xerostomia, as well as other forms of severe dry mouth, such as sjrogens disease, to return to being outdoorsy people again.

I am stuck in a rut spinning my wheels as far as OASSISS©, but I do continue to work at this project, and have attended a number of meetings. As yet I have not managed to get the break needed, this little country girl has not been able to make the right connections with the world of high finance or venture capitalists that would take OASSISS© into production. I am still actively searching for either the right investor interested in an outright purchase or exclusive rights for development. What better place for exposure for a supportive cancer care device than within the pages of a book circulating among those that would appreciate having one the most? I have not succeeded but maybe with the help of the cancer survivor's community we can raise awareness and stimulate the interest or catch the attention of the right person to make it happen?

I would be very interested in connecting with two companies that would like to join forces with the Natural Spring Water Company that is on board. I am extremely fussy about the taste of water, and Callaway Blue not only tastes great, not only is a family founded and operated business, but sampling reports on the water they bottle validate the goodness of the water produced by the natural underground spring it flows forth from. These are the same spring waters that President Franklin Roosevelt believed to be beneficial. Together we continue to search for the right two parties interested in getting in on a low risk low investment ground floor opportunity of a lifetime to produce and/or supply important component parts. One partner would be in Aerosol packaging and the other must be capable of plastics injection molding production with CAD on site. The Lord works in mysterious ways. I'm in the phone book, Hogansville Georgia look me up.

As you can see I have been exploring opportunities, trying to find my niche', trying to get my life back, ever since I finished treatments. Trying and failing and getting back up and trying again. I am sure others go through this as well. It is very frustrating and yes even disheartening at times. I have even begun to feel like it is honestly no wonder others around me are losing faith in my ability to be productive. I have had years and so far I tried an herbal tea business and gave up, I cost Kevin money for a patent that has not paid off and will soon have maintenance fees no doubt and cost more, I keep promising that I can be a published author but up to this point have failed to deliver. I also learned along the way that apparently manners have been left by the wayside in the brick and mortar publishing industry nowadays because no one even had the courtesy to include the standard we're sorry rejection letter. The pages were as crisp and neat as they were when I sent them out, the packages looked as though the contents were moved from the shipping envelope they arrived in right into the SASE included. I thought that was rude, but it was one more thing that made me even more determined to succeed.

DARE TO DREAM BIG EVEN WHEN YOU ARE SCARED. WE CAN ACCOMPLISH ANYTHING WE WANT IF WE BELIEVE IN OURSELVES. NEVER GIVE UP.

It was a comment in early 2013 that ignited the fire that really got me motivated though to come back to *What to Expect When You Are Expecting Cancer* and finish it. Prior to my cancer diagnosis I was involved in programs and after school activities as a volunteer at the small community center near where I live. I had been involved there since the late 1990's, well over a decade. When I became sick I had to stop, and I was away for almost 3 years altogether. I had decided that I wanted to jump back into volunteering. Helping people has always been what makes me the happiest. I started feeling whole again. I organized a new after school program called the Tortoise Pack of West End Center, you can find us online using search keywords "Brick West End Center Mascot", and we also have an active page on "the" major social utility network. We are the Tortoise Pack because I adopted a huge African Sulcatta tortoise named Brick (who has quite the life story of her own) and she is the children's mascot. Our motto is "A Tortoise is never in too much of a hurry to help". Under privileged and/or lower income children often go through periods of displacement, frequent moves and/or go in and out of the foster care system. Brick with her shell is very symbolic for them. I teach "Home is where the heart is and a Tortoise carries theirs everywhere in their community". Doing these things makes me feel good, like my horses do. The group focus has been upon nature and nurturing, compassion and respect for all living things. Animals, Mother Nature and kids belong together. Besides our beloved mascot I have introduced other animals as well, from chickens and goats to horses and rabbits, and the reactions and faces of young children meeting and touching farm animals, often for the first time ever is absolutely truly beyond any value that can be assigned.

Over the past couple of years Tortoise Packtivities at the community center have included; a productive garden two years in row, a feed the hungry food drive during which they collected over 600 pounds of food that was distributed by the Salvation Army, they completed a six week emergency preparedness course led by Brick and Bill E Goat and passed testing and received certificates, we have reached out to Veterans and the elderly, and participated in fund raisers for local good causes, not to mention completing numerous arts and crafts projects, and creating moral story lines where I tell a story with a lesson to be learned and I cannot do it without them because they color the pictures. Brick is on her way to being famous in our small town; her positive message is very popular with everyone she meets from doctors and firemen to teachers and parents. Yes I am exhausted, but it is not the same kind of exhausted from a strenuous or demanding job, we usually only have meetings with activities and projects once a week. I do not earn money, but the reward of those youthful smiling faces when they are proud of something they accomplished together or awed by something new to them? That is priceless. I should probably mention here that while I did manage to hide most of what I spent on activities, it was clear this was just one more thing I was doing that did nothing but cost money. Yes, again I was costing money and bringing none in. This was when innuendos about finances and why was I not working increased. It seemed I was the only one who saw the value of pure happiness.

EVEN IF UNABLE TO WORK WE DESERVE HAPPINESS IN OUR LIVES SOMEWHERE, SOMEHOW. DON'T LET THOSE WHO LOVE YOU, BUT DO NOT UNDERSTAND YOU BRING YOU DOWN.

For a long time outwardly I let the comments roll like water off of a duck's back. Inside though there was a building sense of needing to defend myself. The problem in my mind though was I felt like pointing out my difficulties, what hurt, what makes life difficult, how I "really" felt would be like I was whining or complaining, and I do realize this is the main reason the misunderstanding started that led some to feel I could do more than I was. That and my husband was always bragging about the latest project I had going on with the kids. I love that about him though, he has always supported my volunteering at the center, and now quite often he helps me when I cannot manage something on my own. For example he is the one who tilled the garden plot both years. We both always try to sound very positive when asked how I am doing. I mean who wants to respond to "how have you been?" to someone you do not see often with "Oh terrible I am miserable I spent the day in bed yesterday or I ache all over and my neck is constantly killing me, and my mouth and throat are so dry, etc…" Of course we say "Oh we're doing good" and exchange stories about what we have been up to. They thought I could work because I did not share that I could not. So at least I understood why they did not know what kind of challenges I went through personally. Still on some level, deep inside, I really felt they should just know. It is kind of weird, as years and years pass after the cancer battle everyone but you seems to begin to forget it even happened, and in the meantime we are suffering a slow decline that goes unnoticed.

IT IS NOT WHINING OR BEING A BABY TO ADMIT YOUR LIMITATIONS TO CLOSE FRIENDS AND FAMILY, DON'T TRY TO BE

SUCH A TOUGH GUY, IT CAN LEAD
TO UNNECESSARY MISUNDERSTANDINGS.

I started to not feel good about myself. I was frustrated by my repeated failures to be financially productive, weary of weakness and limitations, my appearance had changed so much since having cancer. I felt like I was a 100 pound scarecrow. I looked like I had aged twenty years and my body felt like it had been more like forty. I continued on with the kids at the center though. I was organizing the 2013 Easter Egg hunt, we were planning and practicing to put on a little show. The children were going to sing a few songs and for the closing they would perform a dance number. I was at the center more often than normal for a couple of weeks in advance of the event because we had to practice. It was during this time that one little sentence pushed me to the point where you dear reader entered my life, I completed this manuscript. The sentence was "If you have enough energy to volunteer at the Community Center and help other people why can't you work and help yourself with finances". I really took this to heart, even though I know it was not meant to be mean.

I do not complain much, I know sometimes I do make it look pretty easy when I am in public and around people, but that is because of the tough guy in me. For many cancer survivors each and every day is a challenge, both physically and mentally, even if we hide it well. Some days when that sun comes shining through the blinds and my body is aching and protesting from every pore I really do just want to pull the blankets up over my head, but I don't. I keep trying, and you will too, it's what we cancer survivors do.

AS SURVIVORS DON'T SETTLE FOR OR SEEK PITY BECAUSE OF WHAT WE CANNOT DO, WE DESERVE RESPECT FOR WHAT WE DO DO.

It really cut like a knife to think that someone perceived me as intentionally or on purpose being lazy or irresponsible or that I was not doing enough or should be doing more to find work. I started researching and found that self publishing options have changed drastically just within the past five years. Now through available online publishing and marketing options it is possible to publish brick and mortar quality books without paying large fees and upfront costs. I would become an author, agent, proofreader, and marketing director. If not for cancer I would never have had the time to accomplish something this big. Everything happens for a reason. It is time to sink or swim.

So here I am Lord and here is this completed book, do with us as you will. My future happiness rest in your hands and the success or failure of *What to Expect When You Are Expecting Cancer; A Stage IVB Throat Cancer Survivor Speaks of Life Before, During and Beyond Cancer* rests in the hands of the dear reader holding and reading it right now. I hope this first edition effort has not disappointed, and is well received, that I have not failed yet again. More importantly I hope with all my heart that each and every reader who finds this book, finds something within its pages that in some small way eases your personal journey through Life Before During and Beyond Cancer. That would make me very happy.

SO IN ANSWER TO THE QUESTION CAN WE BE HAPPY WITH LIFE BEYOND CANCER? YES WE CAN, BECAUSE WE KNOW THE TRUE VALUE OF HAPPINESS.

ABOUT THE AUTHOR

My name is Debra Paulsen, Debbie to my friends, Debster to a select few. I am a baby boomer with an empty nest, which is not intended as polite code for "I am an old lady with too much time on my hands". Au contraire, for my life experiences, coupled with an innate curiosity and diligent research, have resulted in a veritable treasure trove of accumulated wisdom and knowledge, encompassing a broad range of topics. Being an empty nester means that I have the time and freedom at this point to truly devote myself to the issues I find of greatest interest and importance.

I have always been a very outspoken advocate for common sense and decency, and I firmly believe the pen (or the keyboard as the case may be) truly is mightier than the sword. A number of my news blurbs and Opinion/Editorial pieces have published over the years in small local papers. I am a member of the League of American Poets, and *Who Am I* published in the 2007 Edition of *A Treasury of American Poetry III*. Aside from active participation through blogging and social media outlets, I have been a regular contributor, and featured writer for Associated Content (which recently became The Yahoo News Network) for many years now.

I relocated from Connecticut to Georgia in 1998, during my *life before cancer*, and became a well known fixture in the community, attending meetings, participating in events, and through interaction with local organizations. For example weekly trips to The Salvation Army's soup kitchen in Lagrange to drop off eggs and garden produce, and hosting numerous swimming, horseback riding and agricultural focused "fun days" here at our little hobby farm, for the enjoyment of children attending West End Youth Center in Hogansville, and teenagers from Pathways Counseling Services in nearby Greenville

I remained very active in my community until dropping out of circulation for a while to embark upon a new stage in my life, *Life with cancer*. I was diagnosed with stage IVB throat cancer, and my voice was temporarily silenced. I have now entered *Life Beyond Cancer*, with the same heart, positive attitude, and determination that has carried me along thus far. What began as a dream many, many years ago, is now my reality; in the course of my Life beyond cancer I hope to become a recognized and respected voice within the published community.

www.ingramcontent.com/pod-product-compliance
Lightning Source LLC
Chambersburg PA
CBHW072246310526
45795CB00011B/184